Standards for the Management of Open Fractures of the Lower Limb

Standards for the Management of Open Fractures of the Lower Limb

Jagdeep Nanchahal, Selvadurai Nayagam,
Umraz Khan, Christopher Moran,
Stephen Barrett, Frances Sanderson,
and Ian Pallister

Managing Editor: Hamish Laing

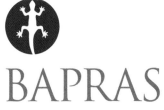

BAPRAS

British Association of Plastic
Reconstructive and Aesthetic Surgeons

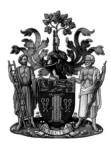

©2009 British Association of Plastic, Reconstructive and Aesthetic Surgeons

Published by the Royal Society of Medicine Press Ltd
1 Wimpole Street, London W1G 0AE, UK
Tel: +44 (0)20 7290 2921
Fax: +44 (0)20 7290 2929
E-mail: publishing@rsmpress.ac.uk

British Library Cataloguing in Publication Data
A catalogue record for this book is available from the British Library

ISBN: 978-1-85315-911-4

Distribution in Europe and Rest of the World:
Marston Book Services Ltd
PO Box 269
Abingdon
Oxon OX14 4YN, UK
Tel: +44 (0)1235 465500
Fax: +44 (0)1235 465555
Email: direct.order@marston.co.uk

Distribution in USA and Canada:
Royal Society of Medicine Press Ltd
C/o BookMasters Inc
30 Amberwood Parkway
Ashland, OH 44805, USA
Tel: +1 800 247 6553/ +1 800 266 5564
Fax: +1 410 281 6883
Email: order@bookmasters.com

Distribution in Australia and New Zealand:
Elsevier Australia
30–52 Smidmore Street
Marrickville NSW 2204, Australia
Tel: +61 2 9517 8999
Fax: +61 2 9517 2249
Email: service@elsevier.com.au

Phototypeset by MTC Manila
Printed in the UK by Bell & Bain Ltd, Glasgow

CONTENTS

FOREWORD

The British Association of Plastic, Reconstructive and Aesthetic Surgeons (BAPRAS) and the British Orthopaedic Association (BOA) have been working to promote the joint care of patients with severe open fractures of the lower limb by plastic and orthopaedic surgeons to minimize complications and optimize outcomes.

The *Standards for the Management of Open Fractures of the Lower Limb* go beyond this to provide an evidence-based approach to improve the management of these uncommon, difficult injuries. The authors have built on the previous guidelines to define the standards of treatment and provide clear guidance of how these patients should be managed. They have addressed all aspects of the care of the patient, from initial assessment through to reconstruction and the indications for amputation. Where there are no clear data, a balanced view of the available evidence is presented, with recommendations based on principles and experience. Importantly, they have also detailed how outcomes can be assessed. I am delighted to note that the intention is for the specialist centres to audit their outcomes using the evidence-based standards. Often neglected are ways to deal with problems when things go wrong, and again the authors have addressed this important area.

The recommendation for the patients to be transferred directly to specialist centres reflects my proposals in the *NHS Next Stage Review* for the treatment of major trauma in specialist centres.

This publication is aimed at improving the quality of treatment through education. BAPRAS and the BOA are to be commended for making the entire publication available online via their websites, free to download in pdf format as well as the abridged version of the principal guidelines. The BOAST poster should enable the Standards to be widely publicised.

Our NHS has been at the forefront of numerous innovations and it is heartening to see that the authors have drawn on a wealth of international knowledge to set the highest standards for patient care.

Professor the Lord Darzi of Denham KBE, HonFREng, FMedSci

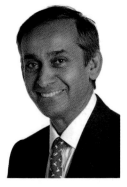

Plastic Surgery is by its nature one of the most collaborative specialties, forming part of many different care teams. No cooperation has been so strong or productive as that alliance with orthopaedic and trauma surgery, and this was underlined in the revolution in the care of the mangled limb, and especially the open tibial fracture. When in 1986 Marco Godina demonstrated how to manage these injuries with the full benefit of the emerging field of microvascular transplantation, he presaged a new era in salvaging limbs. This would not have been possible without the advances in fracture fixation, nor the skills and knowledge in soft tissue debridement and repair. But it has been the synergy between these disciplines and the remarkable cooperation between teams all over the world that has wrought this change most emphatically.

The first UK guidance on the joint management of lower limb trauma came from the BOA and the (then) BAPS in 1993, and this present guidance follows in the same tradition. However now, in a contemporary manner, the guidance is more specific, more comprehensive and evidence-based. These standards will prove invaluable to teams around the world and the joint working party is owed a debt of gratitude from all those managing trauma and all those patients who will surely benefit in years to come.

Professor Simon Kay

President, BAPRAS

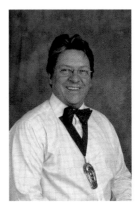

I am delighted to see the publication of 'Standards for the management of open fractures of the lower limb'. This is an excellent example of how the two Specialist Associations, BAPRAS and BOA, can work together to set standards and give practical guidance to surgeons dealing with these complex injuries. I would encourage all orthopaedic surgeons involved in trauma care to ensure that the BOAST and the joint booklet are seen by as wide an audience as possible to ensure that standards of care are improved and assured for the future. The BOA also recommends those wishing to have more detailed information to purchase this excellent book being published from the Joint Working Party.

Clare Marx

President, BOA

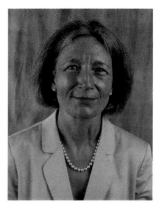

PREFACE

The first meeting between the British Orthopaedic Association (BOA) and the British Association of Plastic, Reconstructive and Aesthetic Surgeons (BAPRAS) was convened in 1991 to foster closer working between the specialties for the management of patients with open tibial fractures. There was a clear consensus that they should be managed jointly and in 1993 and again in 1997 representatives from both associations published guidelines for the management of open tibial fractures. The main aims were to promote cooperation between orthopaedic and plastic surgeons, improve the understanding of these uncommon but complex injuries and encourage their treatment in specialist centres. However, the publication went beyond these, providing an algorithmic approach to the management of the injuries and guidance on 'how to do it'. At a subsequent meeting of the two associations in 2003, it was clear there were difficulties in following the guidelines owing to geographical constraints, lack of resources and remaining areas of clinical controversy.

In 2007, the BOA and the BAPRAS nominated representatives to update the guidelines. An increasing awareness of the complexity of these injuries and an appreciation of limitations of previous classifications to predict outcome prompted the working group to examine the published literature in all areas pertaining to the management of open fractures of the lower limb with a particular focus on injuries below the knee. As in other areas of surgery, there were few randomized trials and an approach based purely on levels of evidence would not have been possible. However, we have been able to draw on a wealth of excellent publications and endeavoured to put the available evidence in context. Where there is no clear consensus, we have drawn on data from associated areas and on our experience. Where no clear choice between available alternatives for management was present, we have tried to provide a balanced view through highlighting the relative merits and drawbacks of each. The evidence base upon which we have drawn is publications in English. We are delighted that the British Infection Society and the Association of Medical Microbiologists have reviewed the guidelines for antibiotic prophylaxis. The format is designed to give the reader easy access to the principal recommendations, which are then supported by details on how they were derived and a bibliography of the relevant literature at the end.

Finally, this publication reflects the current evidence base for our recommendations and we are unanimous in the view that these are the *standards* of care every patient with these injuries should receive. These recommendations should find application beyond the UK.

BAPRAS/BOA Working Party

Jagdeep Nanchahal, Professor of Hand, Plastic & Reconstructive Surgery, Imperial College, London (Chairman)

Selvadurai Nayagam, Consultant Orthopaedic Surgeon, Royal Liverpool Hospital

Umraz Khan, Consultant Plastic Surgeon, Frenchay Hospital, Bristol

Christopher Moran, Professor of Trauma & Orthopaedic Surgery, University of Nottingham

Stephen Barrett, Consultant Microbiologist, Southend University Hospital Foundation NHS Trust

Frances Sanderson, Consultant in Infectious Diseases, Imperial College Healthcare NHS Trust

Ian Pallister, Reader in Trauma and Orthopaedic Surgery, ABM University Health Board, Swansea

Managing Editor

Hamish Laing, Consultant Plastic Surgeon, ABM University Health Board, Swansea

ACKNOWLEDGEMENTS

We would like to thank David Coleman, Simon Kay and Keith Willett for proofreading the manuscript and Mandy Wilcox for compiling the reference lists, as well as Sarah Ogden at RSM Press.

BAPRAS and BOA are also grateful to the following for each making an educational grant to defray the costs of publication and thus allowing the Standards to be available more widely:

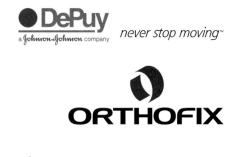

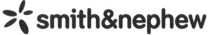

1 SPECIALIST CENTRES FOR COMPLEX OPEN LOWER LIMB FRACTURES

Principal recommendations

1. A multidisciplinary team, including orthopaedic and plastic surgeons with appropriate experience, is required for the treatment of complex open fractures.
2. Hospitals that lack a team with requisite expertise to treat complex open fractures have arrangements for immediate referral to the nearest specialist centre.
3. The primary surgical treatment (wound debridement/excision and skeletal stabilization) of these complex injuries takes place at the specialist centre whenever possible.
4. Specialist centres for the management of severe open fractures are organized on a regional basis as part of a regional trauma system. Usually these centres also provide the regional service for major trauma.

Surgical experience and the development of multidisciplinary teams are key factors in good patient outcome for many conditions, including polytrauma,[1,2] pelvic and acetabular fracture surgery,[3] complex lower limb trauma[4] and arthroplasty.[5,6] Surgical experience usually relates to training and case volume. In the UK, the average district general hospital (DGH), serving a population of 250000, will treat 30 tibial shaft fractures per year and about 25% of these will be open.[7,8] If tibial plateau and pilon fractures are included, each DGH will treat about 60 cases per year and 15% of these will be open. The application of sound surgical principles and evidence-based medicine should result in similar infection and union rates to those of closed fractures; published evidence to date suggests this ideal may only be possible where designated multidisciplinary teams with sufficient case volume and expertise are available to focus on these problems.[9,10]

Severe open tibial fractures with either bone and/or soft tissue loss are less common. Tissue loss may occur directly as a consequence of injury or post debridement. These injuries are high energy types (inferred from the mechanism, fracture and soft tissue injury patterns) and require bone grafts, bone transport and/or flap coverage. Included are the grade IIIB fractures and a 'typical' DGH currently manages two or three cases per year. Multidisciplinary management by experienced personnel, often not available in such hospitals, is needed for these problems.

The characteristics of *open* injuries that should prompt referral to a specialist centre are based on:

1. Fracture patterns:
   (a) Transverse or short oblique tibial fractures with fibular fractures at a similar level
   (b) Tibial fractures with comminution/butterfly fragments with fibular fractures at a similar level
   (c) Segmental tibial fractures
   (d) Fractures with bone loss, either from extrusion at the time of injury or after debridement.

2. Soft tissue injury patterns:
   (a) Skin loss such that direct tension-free closure is not possible following wound excision
   (b) Degloving
   (c) Injury to the muscles which requires excision of devitalized muscle via wound extensions
   (d) Injury to one or more of the major arteries of the leg.

These descriptions reduce the ambiguity that may arise from classification systems which have interobserver variability.[11] If any of the features is noted, it is recommended that such patients are transferred to a specialist centre as soon as the patient's condition allows, and preferably to enable primary surgical management (wound debridement and skeletal stabilization) to be undertaken there.

It is likely that the specialist centres will be organized on a regional basis in conjunction with local trauma networks. In most cases, the specialist centre will also provide the regional service for major trauma.

What constitutes a specialist centre?

These centres require a multidisciplinary team that can deal with all aspects of the management of severe open tibial fractures. The orthopaedic trauma surgeons should have the skill and expertise to provide the full spectrum of treatment strategies for complex tibial fractures, including the various stabilization techniques of internal and external fixation, as well as expertise for bone reconstruction. Likewise, the plastic surgery team will need the expertise to undertake a wide range of local and free flaps. All except the simplest, low energy open fractures require plastic surgical input for the soft tissue component of the injury. Rapid access to theatres is essential to avoid delay in management – the patient needs the right surgeon with the right facilities and with minimal delay.

The specialist centre will need to:

- Include orthopaedic trauma surgery, with special expertise in complex tibial fractures and bone reconstruction
- Include plastic and microvascular surgery, with expertise in vascular reconstruction

- Provide facilities for simultaneous debridement by orthopaedic and plastic surgical teams
- Ensure orthopaedic and plastic surgical planning of management strategy to avoid multiple episodes of treatment, thereby ensuring efficient and optimal patient care
- Provide dedicated theatre sessions for the combined orthoplastic management of the patients during the normal working day
- Include microbiology and infectious disease consultants with expertise in musculoskeletal infection
- Include facilities for emergency musculoskeletal imaging, with angiography and interventional radiology
- Provide a service for, or have access to, artificial limb fitting and rehabilitation for amputees
- Have access to physical and psychosocial rehabilitation services
- Include audit of outcome as part of the care pathway
- Aim to reach a throughput of 30 such cases per annum to maintain appropriate skill and experience levels
- Provide combined orthoplastic clinics and multidisciplinary ward rounds
- Possess intensive care and other trauma facilities for the multiply injured patient.

Timing of the referral

It is likely that with the development of regional trauma networks, many of these patients will be taken directly to the regional trauma centre. However, it is inevitable that some patients will be taken to their local emergency department. These patients should be assessed and the specialist centre contacted immediately. Provided that the patient's general condition permits, transfer to the specialist centre for primary surgical treatment (debridement and skeletal stabilization) should be undertaken as soon as possible. If the patient is not fit for transfer, the local unit should undertake primary surgical treatment according to the guidelines described in this publication, and the patient is then transferred for definitive management as soon as it is safe to do so.

Time is of greater importance in those injuries presenting with vascular compromise. Recognition of this complication by paramedical personnel should prompt immediate transfer to the specialist centre. In the event it is diagnosed at the local unit, immediate consultation with the specialist centre is strongly recommended. Such limb-threatening injuries require assessment and decision-making by consultant surgeons; in some cases a primary amputation may be the preferred option, but the decision is difficult and requires experience.

References

1. Findlay G, Martin I, Carter S, Smith N, Weyman D, Mason N. 2007: *Trauma: Who Cares? A Report of the National Confidential Enquiry into Patient Outcome and Death*. London: NCEPOD.

2. MacKenzie EJ, Rivara FP, Jurkovich GJ, *et al.* 2006: A national evaluation of the effect of trauma-center care on mortality. *N Engl J Med*; **354**: 366–78.
3. Matta JM. 1996: Fractures of the acetabulum: Accuracy of reduction and clinical results in patients managed operatively within three weeks after the injury. *J Bone Joint Surg Am*; **78**: 1632–45.
4. Mackenzie EJ, Rivara FP, Jurkovich GJ, *et al.* 2008: The impact of trauma-center care on functional outcomes following major lower-limb trauma. *J Bone Joint Surg Am*; **90**: 101–9.
5. Khuri SF, Daley J, Henderson W, *et al.* 1999: Relation of surgical volume to outcome in eight common operations: results from the VA National Surgical Quality Improvement Program. *Ann Surg*; **230**: 414–29; discussion 429–32.
6. Kreder HJ, Deyo RA, Koepsell T, Swiontkowski MF, Kreuter W. 1997: Relationship between the volume of total hip replacements performed by providers and the rates of postoperative complications in the state of Washington. *J Bone Joint Surg Am*; **79**: 485–94.
7. Court-Brown CM, Rimmer S, Prakash U, McQueen MM. 1998: The epidemiology of open long bone fractures. *Injury*; **29**: 529–34.
8. Court-Brown CM, Brydone A. 2007: Social deprivation and adult tibial diaphyseal fractures. *Injury*; **38**: 750–4.
9. Naique SB, Pearse M, Nanchahal J. 2006: Management of severe open tibial fractures: The need for combined orthopaedic and plastic surgical treatment in specialist centres. *J Bone Joint Surg Br*; **88**: 351–7.
10. Gopal S, Majumder S, Batchelor A, Knight S, Boer PD, Smith R. 2000: Fix and flap: The radical orthopaedic and plastic treatment of severe open fractures of the tibia. *J Bone Joint Surg Br*; **82**: 959–66.
11. Gustilo RB. 1995: Interobserver agreement in the classification of open fractures of the tibia. The results of a survey of two hundred and forty-five orthopaedic surgeons. *J Bone Joint Surg Am*; **77**: 1291–2.

2 PRIMARY MANAGEMENT IN THE EMERGENCY DEPARTMENT

Principal recommendations

1. Initial assessment and treatment of the patient occurs simultaneously and in accordance with Advanced Trauma Life Support (ATLS®) principles.
2. Assessment of the open tibial injury is systematic, careful and repeated in order to identify established or evolving limb-threatening conditions, and to document limb status prior to manipulation or surgery.
3. Haemorrhage control is through direct pressure or, as a last resort, application of a tourniquet.
4. Wounds are handled only to:
   (a) Remove gross contaminants
   (b) Photograph for record
   (c) Seal from the environment.
5. Wounds are not 'provisionally cleaned' either by:
   (a) Exploration
   (b) Irrigation.
6. Limb splintage is by the most appropriate means of immobilization available in the emergency department. Provisional external fixators are not applied.
7. Antibiotic and antitetanus prophylaxis are given.
8. In addition to two orthogonal views of the tibia, radiographic assessment includes the knee and ankle joints.

Introduction

Open lower limb fractures often are associated with high-energy trauma, and the initial evaluation and treatment of the patient must occur simultaneously. The following steps should take place in every case:

1. Airway with spinal control, Breathing and Circulation managed according to ATLS® principles.
2. Stop external haemorrhage – direct pressure or, as a final resort, application of a tourniquet.
3. Neurovascular examination of the limb.
4. Analgesia if appropriate.
5. Straighten and align limb (if not done prehospital).
6. Repeat neurovascular examination.
7. Remove gross contaminants from the wound.
8. Photograph wound.

9. Cover wound with sterile, moist (saline) dressing and adhesive film dressing.
10. Leave wound undisturbed until patient reaches the operating theatre.
11. Splint fracture (if not done prehospital).
12. Repeat neurovascular examination.
13. IV antibiotics: co-amoxiclav (1.2 g) or cefuroxime (1.5 g) 8 hourly, or clindamycin 600 mg if the patient is allergic to penicillin.
14. Check tetanus status and administer prophylaxis if required.
15. X-ray: two orthogonal views, two joints – knee and ankle.
16. Immediate referral to the orthopaedic team.

Systematic, careful and repeated assessments are important. Neurovascular evaluation of the limb is essential and must be recorded clearly in the notes and repeated after each intervention (e.g. manipulation).

A high degree of suspicion must be maintained for established or evolving limb-threatening situations: severe injuries to arteries or nerves are easy to miss in the acute situation and compartment syndrome can be difficult to diagnose. Capillary return should be evaluated and both dorsalis pedis and posterior tibial pulses palpated. Capillary refill of the skin alone is not a reliable sign. Impaired perfusion raises the possibility of major arterial injury and requires immediate referral. Muscle death starts to occur within 3–4 h of warm ischaemia. Compartment syndrome may not be evident at first check or there may be difficulties in a satisfactory clinical assessment owing to the patient's general condition. Compartment pressures should be measured if clinical suspicion is aroused or if the patient is obtunded.

Active muscle movements must be assessed, but this examination is often confined to movements of the toes or ankle because of pain. Dorsiflexion (common peroneal nerve) and plantarflexion (posterior tibial nerve) should be tested and the possibility of more proximal injury (to the sciatic nerve, nerve roots or spinal cord) considered. Muscle paralysis is also seen with prolonged ischaemia after arterial injury. Appreciation of light touch should be tested on the sole of the foot (posterior tibial nerve) and in the first dorsal web space (deep peroneal nerve). Severe pain on active or passive movement of the toes or ankle raises the possibility of compartment syndrome, but this is difficult to evaluate before the analgesic effect of a simple splint takes place.

A 'mini debridement' of the open fracture in the emergency room does not aid treatment. Digital exploration of the wound is unnecessary, reveals little real information and should be avoided. Lavage through the open wound serves to drive particulate debris further in. Wound management in the emergency setting should be restricted to removal of gross contaminants, photography and sealing. A dressing moistened with normal saline and sealed over with adhesive film is recommended. Antiseptics in the dressing should not be used (see Chapter 9).

Limbs are usually splinted on arrival in the emergency room. A check should be made that the splint is correctly sized, of sufficient length (spanning across ankle and knee) and adequately applied. Slippage may occur during transit and so checks for fit are necessary. If above-the-knee plaster of Paris back slabs are used, appropriate apertures need to be created anteriorly to allow repeated checks of the vascular status.

Antibiotic prophylaxis and antitetanus measures are provided in the emergency room. The recommended antibiotics are co-amoxiclav (1.2 g) or cefuroxime (1.5 g) 8 hourly, or clindamycin 600 mg if the patient has a history of anaphylaxis to penicillin, continued until wound debridement (excision).

Simple radiographs complete the assessment. As with all bone injuries, the two views obtained should be orthogonal to each other and include ankle and knee joints. More than two images are sometimes necessary to obtain a sufficient radiological assessment. Acceptance of inadequate views at this stage is likely to lead to missed injuries and inappropriate surgical planning.

3 ANTIBIOTIC PROPHYLAXIS

(Reviewed by the British Infection Society and the Association of Medical Microbiologists)

Principal recommendations

1. Antibiotics should be administered as soon as possible after the injury and certainly within 3 h.
2. The antibiotic of choice is co-amoxiclav (1.2 g 8 hourly) or a cephalosporin (e.g. cefuroxime 1.5 g 8 hourly), and this should be continued until first debridement (excision).
3. At the time of first debridement, co-amoxiclav (1.2 g) or a cephalosporin (such as cefuroxime 1.5 g) and gentamicin (1.5 mg/kg) should be administered, and co-amoxiclav/cephalosporin continued until soft tissue closure or for a *maximum* of 72 h, whichever is sooner.
4. Gentamicin 1.5 mg/kg and either vancomycin 1 g or teicoplanin 800 mg should be given on induction of anaesthesia at the time of skeletal stabilization and definitive soft tissue closure. These should not be continued post operatively. The vancomycin infusion should be started at least 90 min prior to surgery.
5. Patients with anaphylaxis to penicillin should receive clindamycin (600 mg IV 6 hourly preoperatively) in place of co-amoxiclav/cephalosporin. For those with lesser allergic reactions, a cephalosporin is considered to be safe and is the agent of choice.

Literature review

As with all surgical antimicrobial prophylaxis, an enormous number of studies have been published which include lower limb fractures. However, it is difficult to compare them and to derive a consensus because of different patient populations, the antimicrobial drugs chosen, varying surgical procedures and changes in practice over time. Most studies have examined the role of cephalosporins for prophylaxis and, to a much lesser extent, the value of aminoglycosides (such as gentamicin) and fluoroquinolones (such as ciprofloxacin). There have been three recent relevant reviews,[1–3] one of which is a Cochrane Review.[1]

The very stringent requirements for inclusion in the Cochrane Review emphasize the difficulties of analysing studies in this field. In this review only seven studies were found to be suitable for inclusion and the only clear conclusion was that antibiotic prophylaxis is of proven value in the immediate management of open fractures. No general conclusions regarding which antibiotics, or for what duration, emerged.

In addition to reviewing a number of published studies, the review by Jaeger *et al* (2006) also assessed the national Scottish and the Swedish–Norwegian guidelines and proposed German recommendations.[3] Of note was the lack of international consensus. The authors recommended 24 h of antibiotics following closure of Gustilo grade I and II fractures, and for grade III extending this to 72 h after injury or not more than 24 h following soft tissue coverage, whichever is the shorter. In terms of individual agents recommended for prophylaxis, only cefuroxime was specified. On the basis of a small number of studies, the authors concluded that antibiotic coverage for Gram-negative organisms may be important. In contrast, Hauser *et al*[2] were of the view that coverage for Gram-negative organisms in addition to Gram-positive bacteria was not normally necessary. They were also of the opinion that prophylaxis for *Clostridium* spp was unnecessary and advised against prolonged courses of antibiotics. Again they stressed that when antibiotic prophylaxis is indicated, it should be given as soon as possible, preferably within 3 h. No antibiotic coverage was recommended for low velocity civilian gunshot wounds which did not require open reduction and internal fixation. Open fractures of Gustilo grade I should receive 24–48 h perioperative prophylaxis with a first-generation cephalosporin or similar agent active against Gram-positive bacteria. For grades II and III, the same recommendation applied, except the suggested duration was 48 h. A further option for grade II and III open fractures was a single broad-spectrum agent given preoperatively and extended for 48 h postoperatively. They emphasized that when infections arose, they tended to be with nosocomial multiresistant bacteria acquired during the patient's stay in hospital rather than from the time of injury. When the bacteria from infected fractures were assessed, *Staphylococcus aureus* (65–70%) and *Pseudomonas aeruginosa* (20–37%) were the most commonly isolated, although a wide variety of organisms may be involved, including mycobacteria and fungi.[4,5]

Conclusion

Overall, the available evidence would suggest that antibiotic prophylaxis should be administered as soon as possible following the injury and certainly within 3 h. With regards to duration of antibiotic prophylaxis, Gustilo grade I open fractures should not be treated beyond 24 h and certainly not beyond 48 h. For Gustilo grade II and III fractures, prophylaxis should be continued until definitive soft tissue closure or for a maximum of 72 h, whichever is shorter. This may have to be modified with regards to timing of debridement.

It is more difficult to recommend specific antibiotics on the basis of the published evidence. The best evidence that emerges from this review supports the use of first-generation cephalosporins, of which only cephradine is still available intravenously in the UK at the time of writing. British practice, however, has tended to favour cefuroxime, which has a broader spectrum than cephradine. The use of the second-generation cephalosporin cefuroxime is so well entrenched that it might be difficult to persuade prescribers to use a first-generation cephalosporin such as cephalothin or cefazolin.

At present in the UK, however, there is considerable pressure to avoid using cephalosporins because of the apparent association with *Clostridium difficile*-related diarrhoea, and recommendations promoting the use of cephalosporins may meet with resistance. There is insufficient information on the use of non-cephalosporin drugs in prophylaxis to allow confident recommendations based on observed outcomes. Recommendations must, therefore, be made on microbiological principles, such as a spectrum of activity similar to that of the cephalosporins that have been used. It would be unusual for a patient with a Gustilo grade IIIb fracture to undergo debridement, skeletal stabilization and definitive soft tissue reconstruction on the day of injury. Given that the patient will, therefore, be exposed to hospital organisms over a period of a few days, and that the most commonly cultured organisms are staphylococci (which may eventually include meticillin-resistant strains), coliforms and pseudomonads, the following protocol is proposed:

1. Co-amoxiclav 1.2 g 8-hourly IV or a cephalosporin such as cefuroxime 1.5 g 8-hourly IV as soon after the injury as possible and continued until debridement.
2. Co-amoxiclav/cephalosporin and gentamicin 1.5 mg/kg at the time of debridement and co-amoxiclav/cephalosporin continued until definitive soft tissue closure, or for a maximum of 72 h, whichever is sooner.
3. Gentamicin 1.5 mg/kg and either vancomycin 1 g or teicoplanin 800 mg on induction of anaesthesia at the time of skeletal stabilization and definitive soft tissue closure. These should not be continued post operatively. The vancomycin infusion should be started at least 90 min prior to surgery.

Patients with anaphylaxis to penicillin should receive clindamycin (600 mg IV preop/ qds) in place of augmentin/cephalosporin. For those with lesser allergic reactions, cefuroxime is considered to be safe and is the agent of choice.

References

1. Gosselin RA, Roberts I, Gillespie WJ. 2004: Antibiotics for preventing infection in open limb fractures. *Cochrane Database Syst Rev*; Issue 1: CD003764.
2. Hauser CJ, Adams CA Jr, Eachempati SR. 2006: Surgical Infection Society guideline: Prophylactic antibiotic use in open fractures: an evidence-based guideline. *Surg Infect (Larchmt)*; **7**: 379–405.
3. Jaeger M, Maier D, Kern WV, Sudkamp NP. 2006: Antibiotics in trauma and orthopedic surgery – a primer of evidence-based recommendations. *Injury*; **37** (Suppl 2): S74–80.
4. Patzakis MJ, Zalavras CG. 2005: Chronic posttraumatic osteomyelitis and infected nonunion of the tibia: Current management concepts. *J Am Acad Orthop Surg*; **13**: 417–27.
5. Perry CR, Pearson RL, Miller GA. 1991: Accuracy of cultures of material from swabbing of the superficial aspect of the wound and needle biopsy in the preoperative assessment of osteomyelitis. *J Bone Joint Surg Am*; **73**: 745–9.

4 Timing of Wound Excision in Open Fractures

Principal recommendations

1. Broad-spectrum antibiotics (co-amoxiclav 1.2 g 8 hourly or cefuroxime 1.5 g 8 hourly or clindamycin 600 mg 6 hourly if anaphylaxis to penicillin) are administered as soon after the injury as possible (see Chapter 3).
2. The only reasons for immediate surgical exploration are the presence of:
   (a) Gross contamination of the wound
   (b) Compartment syndrome
   (c) A devascularized limb
   (d) A multiply injured patient.
3. In the absence of these criteria, the wound, soft tissue and bone excision (debridement) is performed by senior plastic and orthopaedic surgeons working together on scheduled trauma operating lists within normal working hours and within 24 hours of the injury unless there is marine, agricultural or sewage contamination. The 6 hour rule does not apply for solitary open fractures.

Literature review

Previous guidelines have favoured wound debridement within 6 h of the injury. The origin of this '6 h rule' remains unclear. It is often quoted but is largely unreferenced.

Few clinical studies have reported a benefit of debridement within 6 h of injury. When studying 56 open fractures in children, Kreder and Armstrong[1] found that the infection rate of those debrided in under 6 h was 12% compared to 25% in those debrided beyond 6 h. Kindsfater and Jonassen[2] reported increased complications in adults debrided after 5 h, although 17 of the 22 Gustilo grade III fractures were in the latter group.

All other reported studies have not found a relationship between timing of debridement and outcome, especially infection. Harley et al[3] found no increase in deep infection or non-union rate in patients who underwent debridement up to 13 h after the injury. The strongest predictor of deep infection was the grade of fracture. Patzakis and Wilkins[4] found that delay in debridement beyond 12 h did not affect infection rate. They found that the most important factor in reducing infection was the administration of broad-spectrum antibiotics. Ashford et al[5] found that delays between 6 and 37 h were in fact associated with a lower infection rate (11% compared to 17% in those debrided within 6 h). Naique et al[6] also found no increase in infection in those debrided between 6 and 24 h compared to those debrided within 6 h. The LEAP

Group reported on 156 grade III open fractures in a multicentre study and found that delays over 6 h and up to 24 h had no effect on outcomes, including infection, time to union, non-union rates, number of surgical procedures, admissions, time in hospital, time to weight bearing, walking speed and time to return to work.[7] More recently Reuss and Cole[8] found no relationship between those debrided within 6 h and those debrided up to 48 h and deep infection. Patients requiring multiple debridements were more likely to develop infection. Following a review of the literature, Crowley et al[9] concluded that the 6 h rule should be re-evaluated and they recommended that debridement of open fractures should occur at the earliest opportunity that experienced orthopaedic and plastic surgeons are available.

Conclusion

There appears to be no advantage to debriding open fractures within 6 h of the injury. We recommend that the wound excision is performed by senior orthopaedic and plastic surgeons on a semi-elective basis. This should be done on a routine trauma emergency list within 24 h of injury. Immediate surgery should be undertaken only if there is gross contamination, devascularization of the limb, compartment syndrome or other injury that requires it.

References

1. Kreder HJ, Armstrong P. A review of open tibia fractures in children. 1995: *J Pediatr Orthop*; **15**: 482–8.
2. Kindsfater K, Jonassen EA. 1995: Osteomyelitis in grade II and III open tibia fractures with late debridement. *J Orthop Trauma*; **9**: 121–7.
3. Harley BJ, Beaupre LA, Jones CA, Dulai SK, Weber DW. 2002: The effect of time to definitive treatment on the rate of nonunion and infection in open fractures. *J Orthop Trauma*; **16**: 484–90.
4. Patzakis MJ, Wilkins J. Factors influencing infection rate in open fracture wounds. 1989: *Clin Orthop Relat Res*; **243**: 36–40.
5. Ashford RU, Mehta JA, Cripps R. 2004: Delayed presentation is no barrier to satisfactory outcome in the management of open tibial fractures. *Injury*; **35**: 411–6.
6. Naique SB, Pearse M, Nanchahal J. 2006: Management of severe open tibial fractures: The need for combined orthopaedic and plastic surgical treatment in specialist centres. *J Bone Joint Surg Br*; **88**: 351–7.
7. Webb LX, Bosse MJ, Castillo RC, MacKenzie EJ. 2007: Analysis of surgeon-controlled variables in the treatment of limb-threatening type-III open tibial diaphyseal fractures. *J Bone Joint Surg Am*; **89**: 923–8.
8. Reuss BL, Cole JD. Effect of delayed treatment on open tibial shaft fractures. 2007: *Am J Orthop*; **36**: 215–20.
9. Crowley DJ, Kanakaris NK, Giannoudis PV. 2007: Irrigation of the wounds in open fractures. *J Bone Joint Surg Br*; **89**: 580–5.

5 GUIDELINES FOR WOUND DEBRIDEMENT (EXCISION)

Principal recommendations

1. Early, accurate debridement of the traumatic wound is the most important surgical procedure in the management of open lower limb fractures.
2. Debridement means excision of all devitalized tissue (except neurovascular bundles).
3. Traumatic wounds are excised comprehensively and systematically and the following sequence is followed in all cases:
   (a) Initially, the limb is washed with a soapy solution and a tourniquet is applied
   (b) The limb is then 'prepped' with an alcoholic chlorhexidine solution, avoiding contact of the antiseptic with the open wound and pooling under the tourniquet
   (c) Soft tissue debridement/excision is safely performed under tourniquet control, especially in cases of extensive degloving. This allows identification of key structures such as neurovascular bundles, which may be displaced, and permits accurate examination of tissues by avoiding blood-staining
   (d) Visualization of the deeper structures is facilitated by wound extensions along the fasciotomy lines (see Chapter 13)
   (e) The tissues are assessed systematically in turn, from superficial to deep (skin, fat, muscle, bone) and from the periphery to the centre of the wound. Non-viable skin, fat, muscle and bone are excised
   (f) At this stage the injury can be classified and definitive reconstruction planned jointly by the senior members of the orthopaedic and plastic surgical team
   (g) If definitive skeletal and soft tissue reconstruction is not to be undertaken in a single stage, then a vacuum foam dressing (or antibiotic bead pouch if there is significant segmental bone loss) is applied until definitive surgery is performed.

In 1917 the Inter-Allied Surgical Conference agreed on the debridement of war wounds. It was recommended that the skin margins be excised, that there should be generous extension of wounds with exploration through all layers, and excision of damaged muscle. These guidelines for debridement of traumatic wounds proved effective during the Second World War.[1] What was practised was a variable combination of excising some components of the traumatized tissues and conserving others. Fackler *et al*[2] compared open drainage versus wound excision in ballistic limb wounds and found that excision promoted quick recovery, particularly when the wound was produced by high energy transfer. Thus, the original guidelines for dealing with war wounds form the basis of current civilian practice.

The term excision may be preferred to debridement as it describes the need to remove rather than debride, which is derived from the word to unbridle (release) tissues.[3] The term excision of devitalized structures was originally used as guidance for military surgeons.[4]

The objectives of debridement are to produce a wound and fracture environment as close as possible to the local conditions encountered in closed fracture surgery. It is the first and perhaps most important step in the effort to achieve infection rates not significantly different from those in closed injuries.

Preparing the limb

Early debridement or wound excision by experienced surgeons holds the key to preventing deep infection in open fractures. After induction of anaesthesia, the limb is cleaned (preferably in the anaesthetic room) using a soap solution and soft brush as a 'social' wash.[5,6] This removes particulate debris on the surface of the limb. The patient is then transferred to the operating room and the limb prepped and draped in the standard manner. An antiseptic skin preparation solution is applied over the entire limb with care taken to avoid contact with the exposed tissues if the solution is alcohol based. Alternatively, aqueous antiseptic solutions can be used.

Tourniquet use during wound excision is a point of contention. Ischaemia and reperfusion associated with a prolonged period of tourniquet use induces the release of vasopressive agents, which theoretically may have a detrimental effect on subsequent tissue transfer.[7] In cases with multiplanar degloving and where the anatomy has been distorted, there is a high risk of injury to the neurovascular structures during wound excision, and here a bloodless field is helpful. In contrast, where there has not been extensive disruption of the soft tissue, excision with the tourniquet applied (but not inflated) may be preferred – bleeding can be a useful sign of viability of the integument and deeper structures.

Tissue assessment

The tissues are then assessed in turn, superficial to deep. Skin is relatively resilient but is vulnerable to torsion/avulsion injuries, which lead to degloving in a plane superficial to the deep fascia and disruption of the septocutaneous and musculocutaneous perforating vessels. Crushing injuries lead to direct devitalization. In cases of extensive flap lacerations, care must be taken to ensure that as much of the integument as possible is preserved, although all non-viable skin must be excised.

The blood supply to the subcutaneous fat is relatively vulnerable and the zone of fat necrosis is often more extensive than that of the overlying skin. Extension of the wounds along fasciotomy lines (see Figures 13.1 and 13.2) allows for access to and excision of the subcutaneous fat as necessary.

An important concept when assessing the wound is that of the 'zone of injury'.[8] This was originally proposed for skin burns,[9] when it was suggested that the area of initial full-thickness skin loss can extend over time. This concept is useful in open lower limb fractures as it highlights that tissues not immediately apparent from external view may be damaged, and emphasizes the need for inspection of the deeper tissues via appropriate wound extensions. It is also useful in planning soft tissue reconstruction, as local flaps should be based on perforators outside the zone of injury and the anastomoses for free flaps ideally should also be placed outside this zone.

Devitalized muscle may be difficult to assess, especially in cases of multiplanar degloving. The four 'C's should be looked for:[10] colour (pink not blue), contraction, consistency (devitalized muscle tears in the forceps during retraction) and capacity to bleed. It is important to inspect the muscle groups behind the tibia as the fractured bone ends are often driven posteriorly and devitalized muscle fragments may be lodged in the medullary canal.

There will be occasions when the soft tissue damage is difficult to assess. A second-look should be undertaken 24–48 h later. However, multiple serial debridement has been shown to be associated with worse outcomes[11] and is unnecessary.

At the end of wound excision the wound bed should approach elective surgical conditions whenever possible, allowing the insertion of internal fixation if appropriate, followed by flap closure.

References

1. Trueta J. 1943: *The Principles and Practice of War Surgery, with Reference to the Biological Method of the Treatment of War Wounds and Fractures.* St Louis: C. V. Mosby, 1–441.
2. Fackler ML, Breteau JP, Courbil LJ, Taxit R, Glas J, Fievet JP. 1989: Open wound drainage versus wound excision in treating the modern assault rifle wound. *Surgery*; **105**: 576–84.
3. Reichert FL. 1928: The historical development of the procedure termed debridement: Pierre Joseph Desault. *Bull John Hopkins Hosp*; **42**: 93–104.
4. Bowyer G. 2006: Debridement of extremity war wounds. *J Am Acad Orthop Surg*; **14** (Suppl): S52–6.
5. Anglen JO, Apostoles S, Christensen G, Gainor B. 1994: The efficacy of various irrigation solutions in removing slime-producing Staphylococcus. *J Orthop Trauma*; **8**: 390–6.
6. Anglen JO. 2001: Wound irrigation in musculoskeletal injury. *J Am Acad Orthop Surg*; **9**: 219–26.
7. Jokuszies A, Jansen V, Lahoda LU, Steinau HU, Vogt PM. 2005: [Plasma concentration of endothelin-1 after myocutaneous latissimus dorsi-transplantation – role in reperfusion injury]. *Handchir Mikrochir Plast Chir*; **37**: 193–201.
8. Yaremchuk MJ, Gan BS. 1996: Soft tissue management of open tibia fractures. *Acta Orthop Belg*; **62** (Suppl 1): 188–92.
9. Jackson DM. 1953: The diagnosis of the depth of burning. *Br J Surg*; **40**: 588–96.
10. Sculley RE, Artz CP, Sako V. 1956: An evaluation of the surgeon criteria for determining viability of muscle during debridement. *Arch Surg*; **73**: 1031–5.
11. Park SH, Silva M, Bahk WJ, McKellop H, Lieberman JR. 2002: Effect of repeated irrigation and debridement on fracture healing in an animal model. *J Orthop Res*; **20**: 1197–204.

6 BONE EXPOSURE, DECONTAMINATION AND PRESERVATION: DEBRIDEMENT

Principal recommendations

1. Extension of the traumatic wound is along the nearest fasciotomy incision (see Chapter 13).
2. Whilst a bloodless field during soft tissue debridement may be helpful, deflating the tourniquet before bone debridement allows satisfactory confirmation of a 'capacity of the bone ends to bleed'. This is probably the most useful determinant of bone viability.
3. Careful surgical delivery of bone ends through the wound extension aids circumferential assessment.
4. Particulate foreign matter is removed with periodic irrigation to keep clear visibility of the surgical field.
5. Loose fragments of bone which fail the 'tug test' are removed.
6. Fracture ends and larger fragments which fail to demonstrate signs of viability are removed.
7. Major articular fragments are preserved as long as they can be reduced and fixed with absolute stability.
8. Lavage follows once a clean wound is obtained by a meticulous zone-by-zone debridement.
9. High pressure pulsatile lavage is not recommended.

Introduction

The environment and mechanism of injury will determine the pattern of open fracture. This information, in addition to knowledge of the type of clothing worn by the patient, should alert the surgeon to the possibility of gross contamination. The exposed soft tissues within the wound may be clean, contaminated or dirty, as may be the bone. An open tibial fracture sustained in a fall on the stairs at home will have an entirely different bacterial load to a similar fracture sustained in a waste land-fill site.

The *contents* of the wound are not apparent from inspection. Elastic recoil of the tissues and first aid measures to realign and splint the limb may result in exposed bone returning to within the wound, carrying dirt and other material with it. Alternatively, the bone end which has burst through skin may be stuck fast with unrelenting pressure on the wound edges and be at risk of drying out.

Wound extension

An adequate assessment and debridement can only be accomplished with suitable exposure of the fracture surfaces and the surrounding soft tissue envelope – access is through wound extensions. Rarely is the wound created at the time of injury sufficient in size or appropriate in location to allow an adequate assessment. Extension of the traumatic wound is along the line of a fasciotomy incision. If the wound does not reach a fasciotomy line, it is first extended to the nearest fasciotomy line and then developed along that line. This preserves the fasciocutaneous perforator vessels that supply angiosomes of skin on medial and lateral sides of the pretibial surface. These, if preserved, may allow local fasciocutaneous flaps to be raised to cover exposed bone at the fracture site (see Figures 13.1 and 13.2).

Delivery of fracture ends

Wound extensions permit the next step to be performed safely – the delivery of bone ends through the wound. It is a common misunderstanding to think that wound extensions and fracture delivery from within increase the extent of damage. Much of the soft tissue stripping was created by the violence of the original injury. Careful surgical delivery of the bone ends through wound extensions will add no further damage provided care is taken to avoid further periosteal stripping through injudicious use of retractors, clamps, etc.

Debridement

Visible dirt and particulate debris should be removed using forceps, curettage, a scrubbing brush or occasionally bone nibblers (if dirt is embedded within the bone). A zone-by-zone approach, using anatomical boundaries as a guide (e.g. layer-by-layer or compartment-by-compartment) encourages a comprehensive assessment. The process is interrupted with periodic irrigation and suction to maintain visibility. Loose fragments which dislodge or separate easily by applying a steady and increasing pull – indicating tenuous or no soft tissue attachments (i.e. which fail the 'tug test') – should be removed. Larger fragments should be inspected for fracture edge or cortical bleeding. If this is uncertain, a hypodermic needle inserted into the soft tissue attachment of the fragment should produce bleeding; if not, the fragment may have a structural soft tissue attachment but without a blood supply, and is likely to become necrotic. It is best removed. Fracture fragments cannot be regarded as bone graft. Necrotic fragments and avascular fracture ends do not contribute to fracture union and serve only as a nidus for infection.

The exceptions to this general rule are those fragments of bone with areas of articular cartilage large enough to contribute to articular stability. Such fragments should be thoroughly cleaned with scrubbing, curettage and lavage prior to reduction and fixation with absolute stability. If absolute stability cannot be achieved, the bone fragment will not revascularize and risks becoming a focus of infection.

Assessing viability of bone improves with practice. Capacity to bleed – seen as a punctuate ooze in viable fracture ends and exposed cortical surfaces (the 'paprika sign') – is helpful but the extent of periosteal stripping and quality of fascial/soft tissue connections also contribute. It is important that bleeding from the medullary canal is not mistaken for viability from a stripped fracture end. In general, non-viable bone fragments, or those of doubtful viability, should be removed. It may also be appropriate to resect non-viable fracture ends until bleeding bone is seen. It follows that assessment of viability is best accomplished without use of a tourniquet. Whilst a tourniquet may be applied to facilitate accurate dissection of soft tissues, whether in debridement or in subsequent flap reconstruction, the ischaemic period induced during surgery should be kept to a minimum and, certainly, bone debridement is better performed *without* a bloodless field.

Lavage

Lavage is not a substitute for meticulous removal of particulate foreign material and non-viable bone and soft tissue. Lavage should begin after the wound appears clean. The type of irrigation solution and the method of delivery remain controversial. A recent review has recommended the use of normal saline and raised concern about the use of high pressure pulse lavage.[1] Although this is effective at clearing surface contamination of bone, inoculation of dirt and bacteria into the soft tissues and bone have been demonstrated, along with damage to the microarchitecture of the bone itself.[2,3] In animal models these effects are detrimental to bone healing.[4,5] Bacterial seeding in the human tibia has also been demonstrated with high pressure pulse lavage, with peak counts in the medulla 2–3 cm away from an osteotomy site. Low pressure lavage (< 14 psi) used early after wound inoculation has been shown to be most effective in human tibial models and complex limb injury models in goats.[6,7] Cleansing human metaphyseal bone with a surgical scrubbing brush has been shown to be as effective as high pressure pulse lavage, but without the risk of iatrogenic seeding.[8] The addition of antiseptics, soap or antibiotics to the lavage fluid has not been shown to add any advantages but does carry the small risk of anaphylaxis for the latter.[1,9]

We recommend low pressure lavage with large volumes of warm saline to complete the debridement of the bone.

Conclusion

Adequate bone debridement is reliant upon the surgical exposure and delivery of the bone ends to enable removal of particulate foreign material and a complete assessment of bone and soft tissue viability. Lavage is not a substitute for debridement and should only follow after an adequate surgical removal of contaminants and devitalized tissue is performed.

References

1. Crowley DJ, Kanakaris NK, Giannoudis PV. 2007: Irrigation of the wounds in open fractures. *J Bone Joint Surg Br*; **89**: 580–5.
2. Bhandari M, Schemitsch EH, Adili A, Lachowski RJ, Shaughnessy SG. 1999: High and low pressure pulsatile lavage of contaminated tibial fractures: An *in vitro* study of bacterial adherence and bone damage. *J Orthop Trauma*; **13**: 526–33.
3. Hassinger SM, Harding G, Wongworawat MD. 2005: High-pressure pulsatile lavage propagates bacteria into soft tissue. *Clin Orthop Relat Res*; **439**: 27–31.
4. Adili A, Bhandari M, Schemitsch EH. 2002: The biomechanical effect of high-pressure irrigation on diaphyseal fracture healing in vivo. *J Orthop Trauma*; **16**: 413–7.
5. Dirschl DR, Duff GP, Dahners LE, Edin M, Rahn BA, Miclau T. 1998: High pressure pulsatile lavage irrigation of intraarticular fractures: Effects on fracture healing. *J Orthop Trauma*; **12**: 460–3.
6. Bhandari M, Adili A, Lachowski RJ. 1998: High pressure pulsatile lavage of contaminated human tibiae: An in vitro study. *J Orthop Trauma*; **12**: 479–84.
7. Owens BD, Wenke JC. 2007: Early wound irrigation improves the ability to remove bacteria. *J Bone Joint Surg Am*; **89**: 1723–6.
8. Kalteis T, Lehn N, Schroder HJ, *et al*. 2005: Contaminant seeding in bone by different irrigation methods: An experimental study. *J Orthop Trauma*; **19**: 591–6.
9. Anglen JO. 2005: Comparison of soap and antibiotic solutions for irrigation of lower-limb open fracture wounds. A prospective, randomized study. *J Bone Joint Surg Am*; **87**: 1415–22.

7 DEGLOVING

Principal recommendations

1. Degloving of the limb occurs in the plane superficial to the deep fascia and the extent of injury is often underestimated.
2. Thrombosis of the subcutaneous veins usually indicates the need to excise the overlying skin.
3. Circumferential degloving often indicates that the involved skin is not viable.
4. In severe injuries, multiplanar degloving can occur, with variable involvement of individual muscles and these may be stripped from the bone. Under these circumstances, a second look may be necessary to ensure that all the non-viable tissues have been excised prior to definitive reconstruction within 7 days.

Literature review

Degloving injuries have been recognized since the 1930s.[1] The forces leading to these injuries include torsion, crush and avulsion.

The viability of the degloved tissues can be difficult to assess and grading systems, based on the degree of injury to the subcutaneous veins, have been devised to help decide how best to salvage the affected tissues.[2] Intra- and sub-dermal thrombosis manifests as 'fixed-staining'. This refers to the state of the skin on clinical inspection where there is a spectrum of discolouration of the skin. The colour can vary from red to blue but fails to blanch on digital pressure. Intravenous fluorescein[3] may delineate non-viable tissues more accurately but requires specialized equipment, caries a risk of anaphylaxis and has poor specificity.

Four patterns of degloving have been proposed[4]:

1. Localized degloving
2. Non-circumferential single plane degloving
3. Single plane circumferential degloving
4. Circumferential and multiplanar degloving.

Over bony prominences, such as malleoli and condyles, pattern 1 can be associated with soft tissue loss, because the mechanism of injury which usually causes degloving in these areas can result in tissue abrasion and avulsion. Although theoretically patterns 2, 3 and 4 can present as closed injuries, in practice, pattern 4 usually presents as an open wound. Circumferentially degloved skin rarely survives.

The degloved skin can be used as a source of skin graft if it has not been directly traumatized.[5] Clearly this can only be entertained if there are no underlying exposed fractures. Extensive areas of degloving without underlying exposed fractures can be covered with widely meshed split thickness autograft with overlying allograft[6] or with an underlying dermal substitute such as Integra.[7]

Conclusion

All non-viable degloved tissues must be excised, especially in the presence of open fractures. The margin of excision can be difficult to determine. Fixed staining and thrombosis of the subcutaneous veins are indicative of skin which will not survive. Circumferentially degloved skin does not survive and the patient with multiplanar degloving should undergo meticulous, systematic excision of all the non-viable muscle. A second look procedure may be necessary 24–48 h later.

References

1. McCollum DW. 1938: Wringer arm a report of 26 cases. *N Engl J Med*; **218**: 549–54.
2. Waikakul S. 1997: Revascularisation of degloving injuries of the limb. *Injury*; **28**: 271–4.
3. McGrouther DA, Sully L. 1980: Degloving injuries of the limbs: long-term review and management based on whole-body fluorescence. *Br J Plast Surg*; **33**: 9–24.
4. Arnez ZM. 2009: Personal communication.
5. Jeng SF, Hsieh CH, Kuo YR, Wei FC. 2004: Technical refinement in the management of circumferentially avulsed skin of the leg. *Plast Reconstr Surg*; **114**: 1225–7.
6. Kim EK, Hong JP. 2007: Efficacy of negative pressure therapy to enhance take of 1-stage allodermis and a split-thickness graft. *Ann Plast Surg*; **58**: 536–40.
7. Violas P, Abid A, Darodes P, Galinier P, de Gauzy JS, Cahuzac JP. 2005: Integra artificial skin in the management of severe tissue defects, including bone exposure, in injured children. *J Pediatr Orthop B*; **14**: 381–4.

8 CLASSIFICATION OF OPEN FRACTURES

Principal recommendations

1. Accurate, simple and reproducible systems for classification of lower limb injuries facilitate communication between healthcare professionals, assist transfer of appropriate cases to specialist centres and should lead to a treatment plan.
2. They provide a platform for conducting detailed audit of care to ensure optimal management of these patients.
3. The Gustilo and Anderson grading is widely used and is relatively simple, but has poor interobserver reliability and is best applied after wound excision.
4. Other systems, such as the AO system, are comprehensive but best used for audit and data collection of outcomes.

Literature review

Methods of classification

Two principal methods have been used to classify complex limb injuries. Broadly, these comprise limb injury scoring systems and classifications based on grading the severity of the limb injuries. The grading systems focus on the injured limb, whereas the scoring systems also include aspects of the patient's general health. The majority of the scoring systems aim to define an 'amputation' score. Comprehensive systems incorporate aspects of both the grading and the scoring systems. Both the grading and the scoring systems attempt to record various aspects of the injured limb including:

1. Energy transfer (low, medium, high or extreme)
2. Response of the injured limb to the deforming forces during the injury (fracture pattern, soft tissue loss, neurovascular injury, presence of compartment syndrome)
3. Age and systemic response of the patient to trauma.

Extremity injury scoring systems

These scoring systems, although not specifically designed for decision-making, have found favour with trauma teams as a means of helping when faced with a severely injured limb. A threshold score may be used to assist in the decision of whether to amputate or attempt to salvage a severely traumatized limb. Therefore, they have restricted application and are of limited value, as they lack sensitivity.

Mangled extremity severity score

This was based on the skeletal/soft tissue damage, limb ischaemia, shock and age of 25 trauma patients presenting to a level 1 trauma centre.[1] It was developed to identify those patients who would benefit from a primary amputation. In a retrospective analysis of all severely injured limbs, two groups emerged: those who were ultimately salvaged and those who required amputation. The mean scores for these two groups were found to be significantly different. A score of 7 or greater was proposed as being predictive for amputation. However, there are limitations to the scoring system because factors such as polytrauma, young age or impaired sensation to the sole of the foot were not included. The mangled extremity severity score (MESS) has been shown to be specific but it does lack some sensitivity.[2] Overall, it *may* have a role in helping the surgeon make the decision of whether or not to amputate a severely traumatized lower limb.

NISSSA

In an attempt to address the shortcomings of the MESS, McNamara *et al*[3] proposed the separation of the soft tissue score from the skeletal score and the addition of nerve injury. The acronym NISSSA stands for **n**erve injury, **i**schaemia, **s**oft tissue injury, **s**keletal injury, **s**hock and **a**ge. It was found that when applied to a severely injured limb, the NISSSA was not only more sensitive than the MESS, but also more specific.

Limb salvage index

This index was applied to injured limbs with arterial compromise.[4] Warm ischaemia time together with scores attributed to injured skin, nerve, muscle, bone, artery and deep veins were added to give a total score. All limbs with limb salvage index (LSI) scores of 6 or greater and Gustilo grade IIIC fractures with associated major nerve injury were amputated.

Grading systems

Gustilo and Anderson

In 1976, the team from Minnesota undertook an audit of open long bone fractures, using infection as an outcome measure. The high energy injuries (grade III) with severe soft tissue loss had the highest infection rates. In a subsequent publication,[5] these injuries were further subdivided according to soft tissue loss and arterial injury requiring repair. The system is prone to poor interobserver reliability, especially with inexperienced surgeons.[6] Recently it has emerged that injured limbs are appropriately categorized by this system *after* wound excision.[7] Another drawback of the Gustilo classification is the relative lack of sophistication in the description of the skeletal injury. Despite these limitations, this system is simple and has found widespread application.

Byrd and Spicer

The vascularity of the fracture and the surrounding soft tissues form the basis of this classification.[8] In type I injuries, both the endosteal and periosteal circulation to the bone fragments is maintained and the surrounding soft tissues are relatively healthy. In type II injuries, the endosteal circulation is interrupted but the periosteal circulation is maintained through the surrounding soft tissues. In Type III injuries there are devascularized bone fragments and the wound requires flap coverage, whilst the Type IV injuries require free flap coverage.

This classification lacks sophistication and has not found widespread application.

Comprehensive systems

AO system

The AO group has devised a comprehensive classification, which incorporates elements of both the scoring and grading systems. Thus, the skin, muscle/tendon, neurovascular structures and the skeleton are graded separately. Grading of the fracture seems to be the most unreliable feature of this system. The reliability seems to increase with the surgeon's experience.[9] The AO score appears to allow better prediction of prognosis when compared with the Gustilo grading.[10] However, due to its complexity, this system is difficult to commit to memory, limiting its acceptance.

Ganga Hospital score

This classification system[11,12] aims to combine the best aspects of the scoring systems and the grading systems based on the experience of a dedicated trauma/reconstruction team of orthopaedic, plastic surgeons and anaesthetists. The system allocates scores for injuries to skin and fascia, bone and joints, musculotendinous units and nerves, with added points for comorbidities such as time to debridement of greater than 12 h, sewage/farmyard contamination, age over 65 years, diabetes and cardiorespiratory disease, polytrauma involving chest or abdomen, hypotension and the presence of another major injury to the same limb or compartment syndrome. A cutaneous score of 3 or greater was predictive of complex soft tissue reconstruction and a score of 17 or greater was predictive of amputation. However, it is not clear as to how some of the scoring parameters were derived, e.g. time to debridement of greater than 12 h, and shortcomings of the system have been highlighted.[13]

Conclusion

Currently, the ideal classification system does not exist. The Gustilo system is simple and, despite its limitations, is used widely. However, it should only be applied *after* wound debridement (excision) and ideally by experienced surgeons. For the purposes of audit and database, the more comprehensive AO system should be considered, although it is much more complicated.

References

1. Johansen K, Daines M, Howey T, Helfet D, Hansen ST Jr. 1990: Objective criteria accurately predict amputation following lower extremity trauma. *J Trauma*; **30**: 568–72; discussion 72–3.
2. Robertson PA. 1991: Prediction of amputation after severe lower limb trauma. *J Bone Joint Surg Br*; **73**: 816–8.
3. McNamara MG, Heckman JD, Corley FG. 1994: Severe open fractures of the lower extremity: A retrospective evaluation of the Mangled Extremity Severity Score (MESS). *J Orthop Trauma*; **8**: 81–7.
4. Russell WL, Sailors DM, Whittle TB, Fisher DF Jr, Burns RP. 1991: Limb salvage versus traumatic amputation. A decision based on a seven-part predictive index. *Ann Surg*; **213**: 473–80; discussion 480–1.
5. Gustilo RB, Mendoza RM, Williams DN. 1984: Problems in the management of type III (severe) open fractures: A new classification of type III open fractures. *J Trauma*; **24**: 742–6.
6. Brumback RJ, Jones AL. 1994: Interobserver agreement in the classification of open fractures of the tibia. The results of a survey of two hundred and forty-five orthopaedic surgeons. *J Bone Joint Surg Am*; **76**: 1162–6.
7. Yang EC, Eisler J. 2003: Treatment of isolated type I open fractures: is emergent operative debridement necessary? *Clin Orthop Relat Res*; 289–94.
8. Byrd HS, Spicer TE, Cierney G 3rd. 1985: Management of open tibial fractures. *Plast Reconstr Surg*; **76**: 719–30.
9. Martin JS, Marsh JL, Bonar SK, DeCoster TA, Found EM, Brandser EA. 1997: Assessment of the AO/ASIF fracture classification for the distal tibia. *J Orthop Trauma*; **11**: 477–83.
10. Arnez ZM, Tyler MP, Khan U. 1999: Describing severe limb trauma. *Br J Plast Surg*; **52**: 280–5.
11. Rajasekaran S, Naresh Babu J, Dheenadhayalan J, *et al.* 2006: A score for predicting salvage and outcome in Gustilo type-IIIA and type-IIIB open tibial fractures. *J Bone Joint Surg Br*; **88**: 1351–60.
12. Rajasekaran S, Sabapathy SR. 2007: A philosophy of care of open injuries based on the Ganga hospital score. *Injury*; **38**: 137–46.
13. Kurup HV. 2007: A score for predicting salvage and outcome in Gustilo type-IIIA and type-IIIB open tibial fractures. *J Bone Joint Surg Br*; **89**: 562; author reply 563.

9   TEMPORARY WOUND DRESSINGS

Principal recommendations

1. Negative pressure dressings may reduce bacterial ingress and tissue desiccation as well as avoid pooling of serous fluid.
2. Negative pressure dressings are not used as a substitute for meticulous surgical wound excision.
3. Negative pressure dressings are not a substitute for coverage of exposed fractures with vascularized flaps.
4. Antibiotic impregnated bone cement beads under a semi-permeable membrane are associated with reduced infection rates.
5. These beads are most applicable in patients with segmental bone loss, gross contamination or established infection, perhaps in combination with negative pressure dressings.

Literature review

Following excision of all non-viable tissues, if the soft tissue reconstruction is not performed immediately, the wound should be covered with a dressing which prevents bacterial ingress and avoids dessication. The application of gauze soaked in antiseptic solutions such as povidone iodine does not have the desired antibacterial effect as the povidone iodine is rapidly inactivated by serum at the concentrations available commercially, and there is a small risk of systemic toxicity.[1] Furthermore, repeated dressing changes should be avoided to reduce bacterial ingress.

Negative pressure dressings

Foam dressings with the application of negative pressure meet some of the criteria of an ideal dressing in the form of the Vacuum Assisted Closure (VAC™) device. Defranzo et al[2] reported a series of patients with exposed bone treated by VAC™. Of the 75 patients in this prospective series, not all had open fractures; some suffered from chronic venous ulceration or diabetic foot ulcers. Dressings were changed every 48 h with continuous subatmospheric pressure at −125 mmHg. They demonstrated that negative pressure dressings applied to exposed bone prevented desiccation of the cortical bone. They also suggested that this dressing may reduce the need for soft tissue transfer. However, the evidence for this is not compelling.

the ankle or knee, the principles of achieving a stable construct still apply.[2] Figure 10.1 shows a selection of cross-sections of the leg and the relevant safe corridors for pin placement. For the majority of mid-tibial injuries, a simple anterior fixator assembly will suffice and permit access for most plastic surgical procedures (Figure 10.2a). With more proximal and distal fracture patterns, spanning the knee and ankle, respectively, will provide greater stability and better soft tissue control (Figure 10.2b–d).

Definitive stabilization

Systematic reviews of whether internal or external fixation should be used are hampered by the number of studies of sufficient quality to be included and the fact that older devices (Lottes and Enders intramedullary nails; older external fixator designs) are used in the qualifying studies.[3]

Factors determining choice

Anatomy of the fracture

Fracture patterns are strong determinants of the definitive method of stabilization: diaphyseal injuries with minimal bone loss are suited to locked intramedullary nails; articular fractures are held well by plates. Injuries with significant bone loss, articular fractures with comminution or dissociation at the metaphyseal level, complex multi-level fractures and those with associated ankle or knee joint instability are suitable for circular external fixation.

Timing of definitive cover

Although provisional bone cover can be achieved by Vacuum Assisted Closure (VAC™) dressings or antibiotic-impregnated bead pouches, early definitive cover is preferable. If internal fixation is used, it is important that definitive cover is achieved at the same time. Delayed cover over internal fixation leads to increased and unacceptable infection rates.[4]

In open injuries which, after debridement, can be closed by simple suture of the wound (typically Gustilo grades I and II), internal fixation can be used safely. If wound closure requires a local or free flap and this can be performed at the same time as definitive fracture stabilization, internal fixation can still be used with low rates of infection.[4] In contrast, if provisional external fixation is used and wound closure delayed, conversion to internal fixation should proceed cautiously. Ideally this is done early and with simultaneous definitive soft tissue cover. The risks associated with conversion from provisional spanning external fixation to internal fixation have not been quantified as yet; recommendations of intervals of 5–14 days as being 'safe' are reported, but basic science research has noted intramedullary canal contamination from pin sites being an early phenomenon and infection from one pin site tracking along the canal to reach

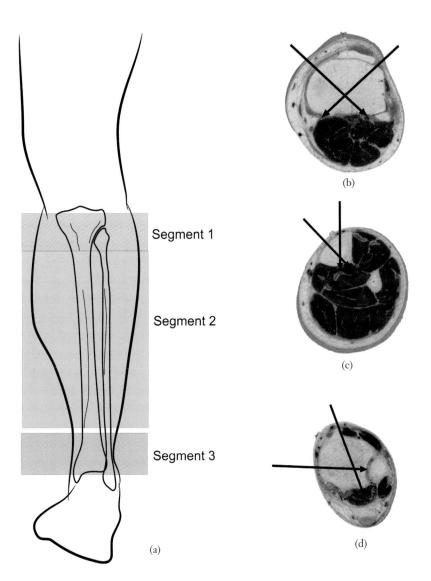

Figure 10.1 Safe corridors for pin placement in the tibia. (a) The tibia can be conveniently divided into three segments in which the safe corridors are relatively constant. (b) In *segment one*, the posterior tibial neurovascular bundle lies close to the midline and directly behind the posterior cortex. Obliquely-directed screws avoid accidental injury. (c) In *segment two*, a 'buffer' of the deep posterior compartment muscles lies between the posterior cortex of the tibia and the posterior tibial neurovascular bundle. Although anteromedial placement is popular, antero-posterior screws are safe as long as care is taken to avoid over-penetration. These sagittal plane screws are useful as they give good access for plastic surgical procedures on either side of the sagittal plane of the limb. (d) In *segment three*, the anteroposterior screw is inserted through a small incision and the plane between the lateral edge of the tibialis anterior and extensor hallucis longus is found. An anteromedial screw is also useful but attention needs to be paid to avoid tethering the medial skin in the event a distally-based fasciocutaneous flap is needed for fracture cover.

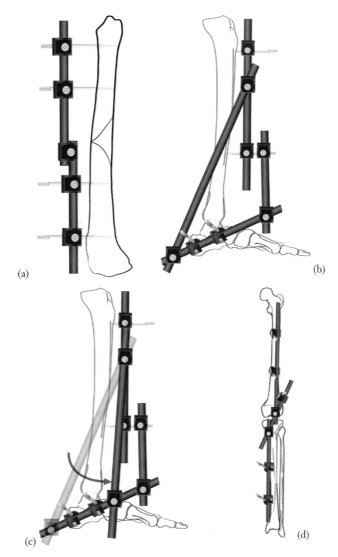

(a)

(b)

(c)

(d)

Figure 10.2 (a) Pins inserted about 1 cm medial to the tibial crest and directed posteriorly allow a simple sagittal plane spanning fixator to be constructed. This provides good access for most plastic surgical procedures. (b) The tibial pins are inserted in the sagittal plane approximately 1 cm medial to the crest. Two coronal plane pins are inserted in the os calcis and neck of talus on the medial side. This arrangement provides good control of the distal tibia by eliminating hindfoot movement. Alternative pin placement includes the base of the first and fifth metatarsals but smaller diameter pins should be used in these areas. (c) Access to the medial aspect of the distal tibia for plastic surgical procedures is facilitated by altering the position of the oblique posterior connecting rod as shown. The rod is returned to its original position after the procedure or the spanning fixator is replaced by definitive stabilization. (d) Control of knee movement (which occurs in the sagittal plane) and access to the front and rear of the proximal tibia are two requisites of the spanning fixator in open proximal tibial fractures. The first is achieved by using sagittal plane pins in both tibia and femur; an additional anterolateral pin in the distal femur significantly improves the stability of the construct. The second is met by keeping the tibial pins distal to the junction of proximal and middle tibia, thereby permitting easy access for potential soft tissue reconstruction using either local or free vascularized tissue.

the remainder of the cavity.[5–8] If conversion from external to internal fixation is planned, we recommended that this be achieved within 72 h of the primary debridement and provisional stabilization (this usually implies that it is performed at the second look procedure), and that definitive soft tissue cover be accomplished at the same time. If this window of opportunity for conversion is missed, consideration should be given to definitive management with modern multiplanar/circular external fixators.

Degree and location of soft tissue and bone loss

External fixation is a better choice if a significant amount of bone loss calls for bone transport techniques. Smaller losses – usually cuneiform in shape rather than segmental, and usually from extruded or debrided butterfly fragments – can be managed by internal or external fixation followed by a planned bone graft procedure.

Degree of contamination

Internal fixation should not be used in injuries highly contaminated with road grit and soil.

Dead space creation and management

In severe injuries, tissue loss occurs either primarily (direct consequence of the injury) or secondarily (as a result of debridement). In both, a cavity is created that becomes a pool for haematoma. Management of this dead space is needed. Techniques include using VAC™ dressings, antibiotic-impregnated bead pouches and, in some instances, acute shortening of the limb with the intention of restoring length at a later stage. Acute shortening, if used for dead space management, may influence the choice of stabilization device.

Conclusion

Spanning external fixation is a convenient technique for achieving fracture stability at the time of primary debridement. If definitive soft tissue cover can be provided for at this time and wound contamination is minimal, internal fixation is a suitable choice for many fracture patterns. If soft tissue cover is delayed, contamination is significant or the fracture pattern is complex with/without bone loss, modern multiplanar/circular fixators are more appropriate.

It is frequently said that internal fixation facilitates plastic surgical procedures. This statement was made when the combined approach to the management of these injuries was sequential rather than simultaneous. In a true combined orthoplastic approach, bone and soft tissue reconstruction strategies are planned together and a decision is made that facilitates a successful outcome in both areas.

References

1. Nayagam S. 2007: Safe corridors in external fixation: The lower leg (tibia, fibula, hindfoot and forefoot). *Strategies Trauma Limb Reconstr*; **2**: 105–10.
2. Giotakis N, Narayan B. 2006: Stability with unilateral external fixation in the tibia. *Strategies Trauma Limb Reconstr*; **2**: 13–20.
3. Bhandari MGH, Swiontkowski MF, Schemitsch EH. 2001: Treatment of open fractures of the shaft of the tibia: A systematic overview and meta-analysis. *J Bone Joint Surg Br*; **83**: 62–8.
4. Gopal S, Majumder S, Batchelor A, Knight S, Boer PD, Smith R. 2000: Fix and flap: The radical orthopaedic and plastic treatment of severe open fractures of the tibia. *J Bone Joint Surg Br*; **82**: 959–66.
5. Clasper JC, Cannon LB, Stapley SA, Taylor VM, Watkins PE. 2001: Fluid accumulation and the rapid spread of bacteria in the pathogenesis of external fixator pin track infection. *Injury*; **32**: 377–81.
6. Clasper JC, Parker SJ, Simpson AH, Watkins PE. 1999: Contamination of the medullary canal following pin-tract infection. *J Orthop Res*; **17**: 947–52.
7. Bhandari M, Zlowodzki M, Tornetta PI, Schmidt A, Templeman DC. 2005: Intramedullary nailing following external fixation in femoral and tibial shaft fractures. *J Orthop Trauma*; **19**: 140–4.
8. Giannoudis PV. 2003: Surgical priorities in damage control in polytrauma. *J Bone Joint Surg Br*; **85**: 478–83.

11 TIMING OF SOFT TISSUE RECONSTRUCTION

Principal recommendations

1. Local flaps are safely performed at the same time as skeletal fixation. Internal fixation is only undertaken if soft tissue coverage can be performed at the same time.
2. Free flap reconstruction is best performed on scheduled trauma lists by experienced, dedicated senior surgical teams following adequate preparation of the patient, including imaging such as angiography or computed tomography (CT) scanning of comminuted fractures. This should be undertaken in a specialist centre.
3. There is little evidence for the 5-day rule. Microsurgery is best performed before the vessels become friable or fibrosed and this becomes increasingly likely after the first week. We recommend that definitive soft tissue reconstruction be undertaken within the first 7 days after injury.

Literature review

Soft tissue cover of a comprehensively excised wound is the cornerstone of achieving infection-free fracture union. Previously, reconstruction of the soft tissue defect in complex limb trauma was relegated to the 'delayed' phase of reconstruction,[1] as the significance of the structures surrounding the fractured bone was not appreciated. High amputation rates were accepted. In 1977, Ger[2] reported on the importance of early muscle coverage of open tibial fractures to prevent deep infection and subsequent amputation. This theme was subsequently developed using free flaps.[3] This large series from a single centre revealed that free-tissue transfer performed within 3 days of the injury was not only associated with improved flap survival, but also reduced deep infection rate. Both upper and lower limb injuries were included and not all had underlying fractures.

Caudle and Stern[4] reviewed the outcomes of open tibial fractures treated with early (within 5 days) muscle coverage. They reported a decreased rate of infection as well as an increased rate of fracture union. In Yaremchuk and Gan's series,[5] the average time to soft tissue coverage of grade IIIB fractures was 17 days. However, serial debridements were undertaken to ensure a healthy bed. These authors reported an infection rate of 14% in a series of patients with large osteocutaneous defects.

Fischer et al[6] considered the timing of soft-tissue cover in grade IIIB open tibial fractures without a bone defect. Early coverage was defined as within 10 days. The other subgroups were those where the open wounds were allowed to granulate spontaneously, those who had soft tissue cover after 11 days to 6 weeks, and those who had soft tissue cover after 6 weeks. It was found that those in the early group spent less time in hospital and had the lowest incidence of deep infection (18%).

Francel et al[7] reported their experience of 72 cases of free muscle flap transfer in open tibial fractures. They defined the early group as less than 15 days post injury, the subacute group as 15–30 days post injury and the chronic group as greater than 30 days post injury. They found that the early group achieved fracture union in a significantly shorter time period than the other two groups. The occurrence of osteomyelitis was also reduced in those patients who were reconstructed early. The major complications all occurred in patients reconstructed after 15 days.

Small and Mollan[8] reported the outcomes of a relatively large series of open tibial fractures treated by a dedicated team. Early coverage was designated as within 72 h. Both local and free flaps were used. Again, the free flap complication and infection rates were highest in those patients reconstructed after 72 h. The timing, it seemed, was a vital factor in ensuring successful limb salvage.

In 1996 Ninkovic et al[9] reported on the 'emergency' use of free-tissue transfer in cases of open lower limb fractures. The definition of emergency was within 24 h of the injury. In this series no cases of deep infection were encountered. Sinclair et al[10] similarly reported a 0% infection rate in their series of open tibial fractures treated by definitive skeletal fixation and soft tissue reconstruction within 72 h. This message is reinforced by the series published by Hertel et al,[11] who compared the outcomes for patients who were taken to theatre on the day of injury and who underwent definitive skeletal and soft tissue reconstruction with a second group who underwent this form of reconstruction at an average of 4.4 days post injury. Those in the early group were found to achieve fracture union sooner, had a lower infection rate and required fewer operative procedures. Crowley et al[12] reviewed the literature on timing of closure of open fractures and recommended early closure, except for heavily contaminated wounds.

The trend towards immediate soft tissue reconstruction was emphasized by the concept of 'fix and flap'.[13] Whilst this system may be applicable in centres with multiple senior microsurgical teams available 24 h a day with access to appropriate facilities, it may be more appropriate for the management of these complex cases by dedicated teams in specialist centres in a more staged fashion when free tissue transfer is required.[14] Delay of soft tissue coverage beyond 7 days in wounds temporarily managed with negative pressure foam dressings was accompanied by a significant increase in the deep infection rate.[15]

Conclusion

The available evidence favours definitive soft tissue coverage of open fractures as soon as possible. This should result in the lowest free flap failure and deep infection rates. However, it is difficult to be prescriptive as to the exact number of days post injury that soft tissue cover should be achieved. Although immediate soft tissue reconstruction, as implied by the 'fix and flap' protocol, may seem to be the ideal, it is best suited to the use of local flaps. We would advocate that complex surgery be undertaken once the patient has been adequately prepared and investigated, and is performed under elective conditions by dedicated senior surgeons working with experienced teams in specialist centres. This is balanced by the technical difficulties as the perivascular soft tissues become increasingly oedematous, friable and eventually fibrotic with increasing time post injury. We would suggest that definitive soft tissue coverage be undertaken within the first week of injury.

References

1. Chacha PB. 1974: Salvage of severe open fractures of the tibia that might have required amputation. *Injury*; **6**: 154–72.
2. Ger R. 1977: Muscle transposition for treatment and prevention of chronic post-traumatic osteomyelitis of the tibia. *J Bone Joint Surg Am*; **59**: 784–91.
3. Godina M. 1986: Early microsurgical reconstruction of complex trauma of the extremities. *Plast Reconstr Surg*; **78**: 285–92.
4. Caudle RJ, Stern PJ. 1987: Severe open fractures of the tibia. *J Bone Joint Surg Am*; **69**: 801–7.
5. Yaremchuk MJ, Gan BS. 1996: Soft tissue management of open tibia fractures. *Acta Orthop Belg*; **62** (Suppl 1): 188–92.
6. Fischer MD, Gustilo RB, Varecka TF. 1991: The timing of flap coverage, bone-grafting, and intramedullary nailing in patients who have a fracture of the tibial shaft with extensive soft-tissue injury. *J Bone Joint Surg Am*; **73**: 1316–22.
7. Francel TJ, Vander Kolk CA, Hoopes JE, Manson PN, Yaremchuk MJ. 1992: Microvascular soft-tissue transplantation for reconstruction of acute open tibial fractures: timing of coverage and long-term functional results. *Plast Reconstr Surg*; **89**: 478–87; discussion 488–9.
8. Small JO, Mollan RA. 1992: Management of the soft tissues in open tibial fractures. *Br J Plast Surg*; **45**: 571–7.
9. Ninkovic M, Schoeller I, Benedetto KP, Anderl H. 1996: Emergency free flap cover in complex injuries of the lower extremity. *Scand J Plast Recon Surg*; **30**: 37–47.
10. Sinclair JS, McNally MA, Small JO, Yeates HA. 1997: Primary free-flap cover of open tibial fractures. *Injury*; **28**: 581–7.
11. Hertel R, Lambert SM, Muller S, Ballmer FT, Ganz R. 1999: On the timing of soft-tissue reconstruction for open fractures of the lower leg. *Arch Orthop Trauma Surg*; **119**: 7–12.
12. Crowley DJ, Kanakaris NK, Giannoudis PV. 2007: Irrigation of the wounds in open fractures. *J Bone Joint Surg Br*; **89**: 580–5.
13. Gopal S, Majumder S, Batchelor AG, *et al.* 2000: Fix and flap: the radical orthopaedic and plastic treatment of severe open fractures of the tibia. *J Bone Joint Surg Br*; **82**: 959–66.
14. Naique SB, Pearse M, Nanchahal J. 2006: Management of severe open tibial fractures: The need for combined orthopaedic and plastic surgical treatment in specialist centres. *J Bone Joint Surg Br*; **88**: 351–7.
15. Bhattacharyya T, Mehta P, Smith M, Pomahac B. 2008: Routine use of wound vacuum-assisted closure does not allow coverage delay for open tibia fractures. *Plast Reconstr Surg*; **121**: 1263–6.

12 TYPE OF SOFT TISSUE RECONSTRUCTION

Principal recommendations

1. All open fractures are covered with vascularized soft tissue.
2. Dressings such as those using foam with negative pressure can temporize following wound excision but are not to be used as a substitute for definitive flap coverage.
3. Relatively low energy tibial fractures are covered by local fasciocutaneous flaps so long as the vascularity has not been compromised by the zone of injury and degloving.
4. Strong clinical evidence to support the use of one form of soft tissue cover over another in open tibial shaft fractures is absent. However, available experimental data would suggest that diaphyseal tibial fractures with periosteal stripping are best covered by muscle flaps instead of fasciocutaneous flaps.
5. Metaphyseal fractures, especially those around the ankle, are best covered by fasciocutaneous flaps, including free flaps.

Literature review

Clinical series: muscle flaps

Fasciocutaneous tissue and muscle are both used for soft tissue coverage in the clinical setting, although the choice between them has been largely based on personal preference. Several authors of clinical studies state that muscle provides superior coverage of open tibial fractures.[1-5] Georgiadis et al[3] highlighted the ability of muscle flaps to reduce both healing time and deep infection, quoting previous experimental evidence.

Small and Mollan[6] reviewed the treatment of 168 open tibial fractures treated over 15 years. They supported their preference for muscle coverage by quoting experimental evidence for the contribution of muscle to fracture healing, with particular reference to its blood supply.[7-11] Further clinical evidence from this retrospective study was used to support the use of muscle, with the highest complication rate reported in fasciocutaneous flaps. The authors concluded that free tissue transfer with muscle would provide the most appropriate reconstruction for the majority of these severe injuries.

Pollak et al[5] reported a prospective multicentre study involving high energy lower limb trauma and the short-term wound complications following soft tissue flap coverage. Rotational flaps, including fasciocutaneous tissue and muscle, were compared to free muscle flaps in 195 limbs in 190 patients. The overall complication rate was 27%, with 87% of these requiring further procedures. Patients in the free flap group had more severe soft tissue injuries, but those undergoing rotational flaps had a higher Injury Severity Score, reflecting more substantial overall body trauma, which may have influenced the choice of reconstruction. Wound complications such as infection, necrosis or flap loss, were significantly higher in the rotational flap group compared to the free muscle group, despite the patients in the latter group having sustained the most severe osseous injury. In fact, patients treated with rotational flaps were 4.3 times more likely to have wound complications requiring operative intervention.

Gopal et al[4] described their 'fix and flap' approach to severe open tibial fractures, with a retrospective review of 84 consecutive patients, which included 79 grade IIIB and five Gustilo grade IIIC fractures, between 1990 and 1998. All patients followed a strict protocol, which included early soft tissue coverage with a muscle flap. Their low rate of infection was attributed to effective management with adequate debridement, skeletal stabilization and subsequent obliteration of the dead space with a well vascularized muscle flap. The same group published data on the outcome and functional status of 33 patients with 34 severe open tibial fractures, of which 30 were Gustilo grade IIIB. With mean time to union of 41 weeks, outcome measures compared favourably to others published for limb salvage and amputation, together with high patient satisfaction. They attributed their success to the introduction of healthy muscle to the fracture site, bringing important cellular and humoral elements to the healing process.[13]

Muscle flaps are thus said to provide excellent coverage for soft tissue defects over open tibial fractures. The plastic property of this tissue, conforming to the defect with elimination of dead space, may be important in reducing haematoma/seroma and subsequent infection. The perceived advantages of higher vasculature and resistance to infection[14] have led to some authors preferring muscle to fasciocutaneous tissue.[15]

Clinical series: fasciocutaneous flaps

Fasciocutaneous flaps have been used successfully in large clinical series to reconstruct open tibial defects.[16–22] The reliability of local fasciocutaneous flaps for lower limb reconstruction was demonstrated by Ponten[24] in his study of 23 cases. The advantages of simplicity, availability and versatility of local fasciocutaneous flaps, replacing 'like with like', offered significant advantages compared to complex microsurgical transfer and sacrifice of a muscle.[16,17,19,24]

Hallock[16] reported on 100 consecutive local fasciocutaneous flaps, which included 67 to the lower extremity. Whilst the majority of patients requiring vascularized tissue had been subject to trauma, it was not clear that all patients had fractures. Major complications requiring further surgical intervention occurred in 15% of patients, with the majority seen in lower limb wounds and attributed to peripheral vascular insufficiency. The coverage of contaminated wounds was highlighted, with short-term healing achieved. This suggested that fasciocutaneous flaps could be used to cover previously infected fractures, challenging the available experimental evidence that muscle was superior in clearing bacterial load.[25] One major benefit of local fasciocutaneous flaps is the relative simplicity of the procedure, and these flaps may be especially suitable for patients with significant medical problems, multiple trauma and higher injury severity scores, who might otherwise not be candidates for microsurgical procedures.

A further study by Hallock[17] compared the relative donor site morbidity of muscle and fascial flaps. This retrospective review compared 147 local muscle/musculocutaneous and 122 fascia/fasciocutaneous flaps to reconstruct all regions of the body, with a total of 45 muscle and 72 fasciocutaneous flaps used for the lower limb. Once again, it was not clear whether all these patients had exposed fractures. Major complications, including nerve injury, failed graft, necrosis or ulceration, were infrequent in both groups, with overall donor site complications reaching 14% in each group. Most difficulties, however, were encountered below the knee with fasciocutaneous flap donor sites, where no local muscle option was available. In this study, Hallock stated that the skin grafted donor sites were cosmetically unappealing.

The role of muscle and fascia flaps in lower extremity trauma was again assessed in a later study by the same author.[19] A retrospective review over an 18-year period provided details of flap coverage in 160 limbs in 155 patients, of which 60 were local muscle, 50 were local fascial and 74 were free muscle and fascial flaps. Flap selection was not randomly assigned, but based on clinical need of the patient. Complications were related to the severity of the injury. There were more complications associated with free flap transfer (39%), whereas local muscle and local fascia flaps had similar morbidity (27% and 30%, respectively). It was concluded that flap selection depended on the location and severity of the original injury and flap availability.

Erdmann et al[18] published their experience of fasciocutaneous flaps in lower limb trauma over a 5-year period. Open tibial fractures in 61 patients were reconstructed with distally based, islanded fasciocutaneous flaps, covering the distal one-third of the leg, ankle, heel or foot. Twenty-five fractures were graded as Gustilo IIIB. The overall complication rate was 7.6%. Five patients had complete flap loss and all of these had been used to cover grade IIIB fractures. Thus, the complication rate for coverage of these injuries with distally based islanded fasciocutaneous flaps reached 20%. The mean time to fracture healing was 5.9 months, with a mean follow-up of 13 months. Chronic osteomyelitis, leading to non-union, developed in four patients.

Evidence for the successful use of fasciocutaneous flaps in chronic osteomyelitis of the lower limb was provided by Hong et al.[21] They described their experience over 3 years in 28 consecutive patients treated with surgical debridement and reconstruction using free anterolateral thigh perforator flaps, although six of the fasciocutaneous flaps were combined with a segment of vastus lateralis muscle. Although coverage of infected defects with muscle flaps is well known, they proposed that where there is little dead space, skin and subcutaneous tissues would provide stable wound coverage. This was achieved in their series, with direct closure of the donor site minimizing morbidity. The well contoured soft tissue flaps allowed effective resurfacing at the level of the ankle, permitting normal footwear. Furthermore, unlike the muscle flap, the elasticity of the skin flap allowed easy re-exploration for secondary bone grafting procedures, with tension-free closure. They concluded that this time-efficient, functional, aesthetic and safe procedure, using the anterolateral thigh perforator flap, provided successful coverage for chronic infection, following adequate debridement and obliteration of dead space, although long-term follow-up was required.

More recently, the sural artery flap has become increasingly popular. In a multicentre review of 70 flaps, Baumeister et al,[26] found that up to 36% developed necrosis, and this was most likely to occur in patients with comorbidity, including diabetes mellitus, venous insufficiency and peripheral arterial disease.

Experimental evidence

Chang and Mathes[14] were the first to undertake a comparison of different tissues in an animal model. A canine infection model was used, with no underlying fracture. Chambers inoculated with bacteria were inserted beneath random pattern flaps raised on the flanks. Muscle was found to be superior in eliminating bacteria from the wound bed. This was attributed to its higher vascularity, giving it greater capacity to deliver blood-borne components of the immunological system and oxygen. The random-pattern fasciocutaneous flaps, however, may have been less well vascularized than fasciocutaneous flaps with an axial-pattern blood supply. Further work by this group sought to refine the hypothesis and compare musculocutaneous and fasciocutaneous flaps.[25] The interface of each flap was studied with respect to inhibition of bacterial growth within wound fluid and this was correlated with cutaneous blood flow and tissue oxygen tension. Although initial blood flow and tissue oxygen tension in the cutaneous portion was higher in the fasciocutaneous group, muscle had increased ability to reduce the bacterial count at the wound surface. Finally, histological examination of the interface of both flaps was performed and this revealed greater evidence of repair beneath muscle, with increased collagen deposition compared to the under surface of the fasciocutaneous flaps. A later refinement to the study utilizing a different method of assessment of blood flow allowed measurements at the flap interface.[27] This showed an initial increase in muscle blood flow in the first 24 h. The deep surface of the fasciocutaneous flap underwent a slower and steadier increase in blood flow over the experimental period of 6 days to exceed that of muscle by this point. The conclusion from these studies was that muscle had some intrinsic ability to suppress bacterial growth within the wound. This was attributed to the initial increase in interface blood flow that corresponded to bacterial elimination, but other factors could not be excluded.

Schemitsch, Richards and co-workers compared cutaneous and muscle tissues in a canine open tibial fracture model.[28–32] A devascularized segment of tibia was covered with either transposed tibialis muscle and the skin incision closed (muscle flap group) or skin directly (skin group). In this series of experiments, several parameters relating to the fracture healing process were reviewed. Segmental osteotomy was found to increase blood flow in the surrounding tissues (skin, muscle), as well as in marrow and tibial cortex.[28] The most notable positive finding in favour of muscle was significantly increased bone blood flow in the muscle flap group compared to the skin group, particularly anteriorly.[31] The rate of osteotomy union was also increased in the group with muscle flap coverage.[29,31]

Muscle flaps were found also significantly to increase cortical porosity, enveloping callus and intracortical new bone formation.[30] There was no direct correlation between the soft tissue blood flow and the indices of bone repair. Resting muscle blood flow was found to be higher in the control limb using the microsphere technique.[28] Subsequent investigation of flap perfusion showed no difference in extraosseous soft tissue perfusion at the fracture site between the different groups.[32] However, the model is open to criticism. Fascia beneath the anterior skin was excised in both groups, creating a muscle flap group and a skin only group. The absence of fascia means therefore, that the clinical situation is not reproduced. Furthermore, only one-third of the circumference of the osteotomised tibial segment was in contact with the soft tissue flap, with the posterior segment in direct apposition with intact periosteum and musculature in both groups. This did not allow exclusive comparison of the two tissues and their biological effect on fracture healing.

In an attempt to overcome the limitations of previous studies, Harry *et al*[33] developed a murine open tibial fracture model. Experimental groups were devised to allow comparison of either muscle alone or skin plus fascia in direct contact with healing bone. In order exclusively to assess the relative efficacy of muscle and fasciocutaneous tissue to promote healing of a fracture stripped of periosteum, a piece of sterile inert material (polytetrafluoroethylene) was positioned anteriorly, excluding skin and fascia (muscle group) or posteriorly, excluding muscle (fasciocutaneous group). Skeletal repair was assessed histologically and quantified by histomorphometry, quantitative peripheral computed tomography (pQCT) and mechanical testing using a four-point bending technique.

This standardized, reproducible model allowed characterization of the morphology of open fracture healing. At 28 days post fracture, there was faster healing in the experimental muscle coverage group compared to skin and fascia alone. Furthermore, there was almost 50% more cortical bone content and a three-fold stronger union beneath muscle compared to fasciocutaneous tissue ($p < 0.05$ by one-way ANOVA). Interestingly, at all time points, there was a higher vascular density in the fasciocutaneous tissue compared to the muscle.[34]

Exclusive comparison of muscle and fasciocutaneous tissue using the murine model demonstrated that muscle is superior for the coverage of open tibial diaphyseal fractures for both the rate and quality of fracture healing.

Conclusion

There are no randomized clinical studies comparing the use of local fasciocutaneous or free flaps. Indeed, such a study would be difficult to undertake as large soft tissue defects accompanied by extensive degloving cannot be covered by local fasciocutaneous flaps. The available evidence would suggest that there are fewer complications with free flaps when performed by experienced surgeons in centres with a large experience, and that the patients traditionally thought to tolerate microvascular procedures least well are also most prone to complications following local fasciocutaneous flaps. These include the elderly and those with diabetes, venous insufficiency and peripheral vascular disease.

Whilst there are no robust data from clinical studies favouring the coverage of open fractures with muscle or fasciocutaneous tissue, animal models provide convincing evidence for the coverage of open tibial shaft fractures with muscle. With the available data, we would suggest that fasciocutaneous flaps may be superior for coverage of metaphyseal fractures, particularly around the ankle. With the increasing popularity of the use of the free anterolateral thigh flaps and the option to raise chimaeric flaps including a segment of vastus lateralis, the division is blurred. Indeed, it may be optimal to use these chimaeric flaps to cover tibial shaft fractures, and this would have the additional benefit of avoiding the unsightly skin grafted donor site below the knee, which accompanies many local fasciocutaneous flaps.

References

1. Byrd HS, Cierny G, 3rd, Tebbetts JB. 1981: The management of open tibial fractures with associated soft-tissue loss: External pin fixation with early flap coverage. *Plast Reconstr Surg*; **68**: 73–82.
2. Fischer MD, Gustilo RB, Varecka TF. 1991: The timing of flap coverage, bone-grafting, and intramedullary nailing in patients who have a fracture of the tibial shaft with extensive soft-tissue injury. *J Bone Joint Surg Am*; **73**: 1316–22.
3. Georgiadis GM, Behrens FF, Joyce MJ, Earle AS, Simmons AL. 1993: Open tibial fractures with severe soft-tissue loss. Limb salvage compared with below-the-knee amputation. *J Bone Joint Surg Am*; **75**: 1431–41.
4. Gopal S, Majumder S, Batchelor AG, Knight SL, De Boer P, Smith RM. 2000: Fix and flap: The radical orthopaedic and plastic treatment of severe open fractures of the tibia. *J Bone Joint Surg Br*; **82**: 959–66.
5. Pollak AN, McCarthy ML, Burgess AR. 2000: Short-term wound complications after application of flaps for coverage of traumatic soft-tissue defects about the tibia. The Lower Extremity Assessment Project (LEAP) Study Group. *J Bone Joint Surg Am*; **82**: 1681–91.
6. Small JO, Mollan RA. 1992: Management of the soft tissues in open tibial fractures. *Br J Plast Surg*; **45**: 571–7.
7. Gothman L. 1962: Local arterial changes associated with diastasis in experimental fractures of the rabbit's tibia treated with intramedullary nailing. A microangiographic study. *Acta Chir Scand*; **123**: 104–10.
8. Trueta J, Buhr AJ. 1963: The Vascular Contribution to Osteogenesis. V. The Vasculature Supplying the Epiphysial Cartilage in Rachitic Rats. *J Bone Joint Surg Br*; **45**: 572–81.
9. Rhinelander FW. 1968: The normal microcirculation of diaphyseal cortex and its response to fracture. *J Bone Joint Surg Am*; **50**: 784–800.
10. Holden CE. 1972: The role of blood supply to soft tissue in the healing of diaphyseal fractures. An experimental study. *J Bone Joint Surg Am*; **54**: 993–1000.

11. Whiteside LA, Ogata K, Lesker P, Reynolds FC. 1978: The acute effects of periosteal stripping and medullary reaming on regional bone blood flow. *Clin Orthop*; **131**: 266–72.

12. Macnab I, De Haas WG. 1974: The role of periosteal blood supply in the healing of fractures of the tibia. *Clin Orthop Relat Res*; **105**: 27–33.

13. Gopal S, Giannoudis PV, Murray A, Matthews SJ, Smith RM. 2004: The functional outcome of severe, open tibial fractures managed with early fixation and flap coverage. *J Bone Joint Surg Br*; **86**: 861–7.

14. Chang N, Mathes SJ. 1982: Comparison of the effect of bacterial inoculation in musculocutaneous and random-pattern flaps. *Plast Reconstr Surg*; **70**: 1–10.

15. Tropet Y, Garbuio P, Obert L, Ridoux PE. 1999: Emergency management of type IIIB open tibial fractures. *Br J Plast Surg*; **52**: 462–70.

16. Hallock GG. 1991: Complications of 100 consecutive local fasciocutaneous flaps. *Plast Reconstr Surg*; **88**: 264–8.

17. Hallock GG. 1993: Relative donor-site morbidity of muscle and fascial flaps. *Plast Reconstr Surg*; **92**: 70–6.

18. Erdmann MW, Court-Brown CM, Quaba AA. 1997: A five year review of islanded distally based fasciocutaneous flaps on the lower limb. *Br J Plast Surg*; **50**: 421–7.

19. Hallock GG. 2000: Utility of both muscle and fascia flaps in severe lower extremity trauma. *J Trauma*; **48**: 913–7.

20. Hallock GG. 2004: Lower extremity muscle perforator flaps for lower extremity reconstruction. *Plast Reconstr Surg*; **114**: 1123–30.

21. Hong JP, Shin HW, Kim JJ, Wei FC, Chung YK. 2005: The use of anterolateral thigh perforator flaps in chronic osteomyelitis of the lower extremity. *Plast Reconstr Surg*; **115**: 142–7.

22. Van Landuyt K, Blondeel P, Hamdi M, Tonnard P, Verpaele A, Monstrey S. 2005: The versatile DIEP flap: Its use in lower extremity reconstruction. *Br J Plast Surg*; **58**: 2–13.

23. Ponten B. 1981: The fasciocutaneous flap: Its use in soft tissue defects of the lower leg. *Br J Plast Surg*; **34**: 215–20.

24. Khan U, Pickford M. 2000: Use of an islanded fasciocutaneous flap in the lower limb following distraction callotasis. *Br J Plast Surg*; **53**: 705–6.

25. Calderon W, Chang N, Mathes SJ. 1986: Comparison of the effect of bacterial inoculation in musculocutaneous and fasciocutaneous flaps. *Plast Reconstr Surg*; **77**: 785–94.

26. Baumeister SP, Spierer R, Erdmann D, Sweiss R, Levin LS, Germann GK. 2003: A realistic complication analysis of 70 sural artery flap in a multimorbid patient group. *Plast Reconstr Surg* 2003; **112**: 129–40.

27. Gosain A, Chang N, Mathes S, Hunt TK, Vasconez L. 1990: A study of the relationship between blood flow and bacterial inoculation in musculocutaneous and fasciocutaneous flaps. *Plast Reconstr Surg*; **86**: 1152–62; discussion 1163.

28. Anderson GI, Richards RR, Paitich B, McKee M, Schemitsch EH. 1991: Soft-tissue blood flow after segmental osteotomy of the canine tibia. *Ann Plast Surg*; **27**: 49–55.

29. Richards RR, McKee MD, Paitich CB, Anderson GI, Bertoia JT. 1991: A comparison of the effects of skin coverage and muscle flap coverage on the early strength of union at the site of osteotomy after devascularization of a segment of canine tibia. *J Bone Joint Surg Am*; **73**: 1323–30.

30. Richards RR, Orsini EC, Mahoney JL, Verschuren R. 1987: The influence of muscle flap coverage on the repair of devascularized tibial cortex: an experimental investigation in the dog. *Plast Reconstr Surg*; **79**: 946–58.

31. Richards RR, Schemitsch EH. 1989: Effect of muscle flap coverage on bone blood flow following devascularization of a segment of tibia: An experimental investigation in the dog. *J Orthop Res*; **7**: 550–8.

32. Schemitsch EH, Weinberg JA, McKee MD, Richards RR. 1997: The relative importance of intramedullary, intracortical, and extraosseous soft-tissue blood flow to the repair of devascularized canine tibial cortex. *Ann Plast Surg*; **38**: 623–31.

33. Harry LE, Sandison A, Paleolog EM, Hansen U, Pearse MF, Nanchahal J. 2008: Comparison of the healing of open tibial fractures covered with either muscle or fasciocutaneous tissue in a murine model. *J Orthop Res*; **26**: 1238–44.
34. Harry LE, Sandison A, Palelog EM, Pearse MF, Nanchahal J. 2009: Soft tissue reconstruction of open tibial fractures: An in vivo study of the effect of vascularity on fracture healing. *Plast Reconstr Surg*; in press.

13 COMPARTMENT SYNDROME

Principal recommendations

1. Compartment syndrome is a surgical emergency and must be diagnosed promptly and treated.
2. The early signs are paraesthesia in the distribution of the sensory nerves passing through the affected compartment and disproportionate pain, especially on passive stretch of the affected muscles.
3. These important signs may be affected by the previous administration of peripheral nerve blocks and regional anaesthesia, as well by the presence of nerve injury.
4. Compartment syndrome does not usually result in the loss of peripheral pulses. Absent pulses should alert the surgeon to the possibility of vascular injury.
5. Intracompartment pressure measurement is performed most reliably using devices designed specifically for this purpose. A difference of 30 mmHg or less between the measured pressure and the diastolic blood pressure is a reasonable threshold for decompression.
6. Every effort is made to achieve an accurate diagnosis because inappropriate fasciotomy can be associated with significant morbidity.
7. The two-incision technique provides optimal access for four-compartment decompression. The medial incision does not compromise availability of local fasciocutaneous flaps. It can also be used to extend pre-existing traumatic lacerations to achieve access for debridement as well as provide an approach to the posterior tibial vessels as recipient vessels for free flaps.
8. All non-viable muscle is excised and fasciotomy wounds either closed with split skin grafts or directly, if possible, once the swelling has reduced.
9. A late diagnosis of compartment syndrome is a management dilemma. Once the muscle is no longer viable, compartment release will predispose to infection and may result in compartmentectomy or amputation of the limb.

Literature review[1]

Acute limb compartment syndrome is a surgical emergency characterized by raised pressure within an unyielding osteofascial compartment, resulting in local tissue hypoxia. Sustained elevation of tissue pressure reduces capillary perfusion below a level necessary for tissue viability and irreversible muscle and nerve damage may occur within hours. The increased intracompartmental pressure (ICP) must be promptly decompressed by surgical fasciotomy. Missed diagnosis and late decompression are associated with significant morbidity due to irreversible ischaemic necrosis of the muscles and nerves within the compartment. Increased awareness of compartment syndrome[1] and the advent of ICP measurements have enabled early diagnosis and treatment. However, some authors[2,3] have highlighted the problems associated with ICP measurements. Furthermore, late or poorly-performed fasciotomies may contribute to morbidity.

The key clinical feature of compartment syndrome in the conscious patient is severe pain, out of proportion to the injury, which fails to improve in the expected clinical time course post operatively and is aggravated by passive muscle stretch. Sensory loss within the distribution of the nerves traversing the involved compartments may be a useful early sign. The diagnosis may be difficult in the presence of impaired consciousness, in children and in patients with regional nerve blocks. Although ICP can be easily measured using readily available devices, there is wide variation in the ICP value that is accepted as diagnostic.[3] The difference between the diastolic pressure and the ICP has been suggested as a more sensitive indicator of tissue perfusion pressure, and a value of 30 mmHg or less has been recommended as the threshold for fasciotomy.[4] However, treatment based on this measurement alone may lead to unnecessary surgery.[3] Increased specificity can be achieved by combining the reduced perfusion pressure with the presence of clinical symptoms, but at the expense of a much reduced sensitivity.[3] ICP measurements are not necessary if the diagnosis of a compartment syndrome is clinically apparent and are probably best reserved for uncooperative patients or equivocal cases, where serial measurements may be required. Continuous monitoring has not been shown to be of any benefit in alert patients who are adequately observed.[5] It is of concern that in the UK less than 50% of hospitals had dedicated ICP measuring devices.[6] Straight needles are less accurate than side port needles and slit catheters. Arterial manometers, IV pumps and the Stryker™ device have been shown to be more reliable than the Whitesides apparatus.[7,8]

Despite the problems associated with long skin incisions,[9] open fasciotomy by incision of the skin and fascia is the most reliable method for adequate compartment decompression.[10] However, performing fasciotomies on a tense, swollen limb can be a daunting and difficult undertaking. We recommend the two-incision technique,[11] as endorsed by the previous joint working committee of the British Association of Plastic Surgeons and the British Orthopaedic Association.[12] The superficial and deep posterior compartments are decompressed through a medial longitudinal incision placed 1–2 cm posterior to the medial border of the tibia. A second longitudinal incision 2 cm lateral to the anterior tibial border decompresses the anterior and peroneal compartments. Accurate placement of the incisions is essential. The medial incision must be anterior to the posterior tibial artery to avoid injury to the perforating vessels that supply the skin used for local fasciocutaneous flaps.[12] However, placement too anteriorly leads to exposure of the tibia and any underlying fracture. Palpation of the subcutaneous borders of the tibia can be difficult in the swollen leg and we recommend marking anatomical landmarks before making the incisions. Care must be taken when decompressing the deep posterior compartment, as the posterior tibial neurovascular bundle lies just deep to the investing fascia. Proximally, part of the origin of the soleus muscle may need to be released from the tibia. A lateral incision inadvertently placed over the fibula will expose periosteum, and extending the incision too far distally may expose the peroneal tendons. Exposure of bone or tendons increases the risks of delayed healing, infection and ultimately, amputation. Following decompression, the muscle viability should be carefully assessed and all non-viable tissue must be excised.

Management of fasciotomy wounds remains controversial. Wound complications were recorded in 51% of patients who had primary or delayed primary closure compared to 5% who had split skin grafts.[13] If all devitalized tissue has been confidently excised, we favour immediate coverage with meshed, split skin grafts secured with a negative pressure foam dressing. If it is considered that the incisions may close directly within a few days following reduction of swelling, then a temporary negative pressure foam dressing may be applied. Cosmesis may be improved by subsequent scar revision.

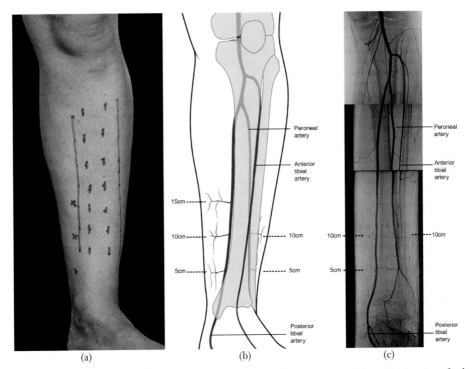

(a) (b) (c)

Figure 13.1 Recommended incisions for fasciotomy and wound extensions. (a) Margins of subcutaneous border of tibia marked in green, fasciotomy incisions in blue and the perforators on the medial side arising from the posterior tibial vessels in red. (b) Line drawing depicting the location of the perforators. (c) Montage of an arteriogram. The 10 cm perforator on the medial side is usually the largest and most reliable for distally-based fasciocutaneous flaps. In this patient, the anterior tibial artery had been disrupted following an open dislocation of the ankle; hence the poor flow evident in this vessel in the distal one-third of the leg. The distances of the perforators from the tip of the medial malleolus are approximate and vary between patients. It is essential to preserve the perforators and avoid incisions crossing the line between them.

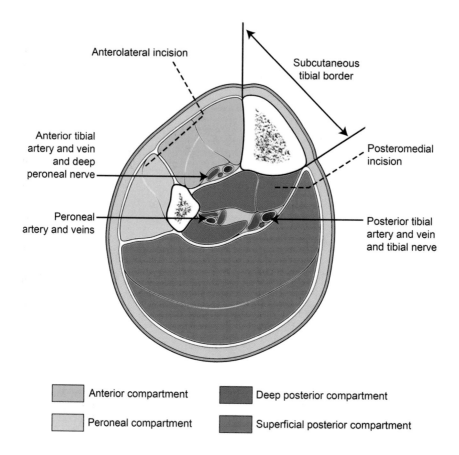

Figure 13.2 Cross-section through the leg showing incisions to decompress all four compartments. The medial incision is situated 1.5 cm from the medial subcutaneous border of the tibia. The lateral incision is placed 2 cm lateral to the lateral subcutaneous tibial border. The lateral dissection continues subfascially until the peroneal septum, which must then be divided.

Fasciotomy is not a benign procedure and there is some evidence to suggest that it may lead to chronic venous insufficiency due to impairment of the calf muscle pump.[14] The role of fasciotomy in late cases of compartment syndrome is questionable, and it has been suggested that release of the compartments in this situation should not be performed.[15] In a review of 31 patients following crush injury treated non-operatively, none developed life-threatening sepsis or required acute amputation.[16] Established myoneural deficits seldom recover following fasciotomy. Furthermore, fasciotomy performed more than 35 h after injury was invariably associated with severe infection and even death.[17] However, the definition of late diagnosis remains unclear and there is evidence that even after a period as short as 3 h, there is evidence of muscle necrosis, although there was variation between individuals.[18] This suggests that acute compartment syndrome may be of varying severity. Patients who undergo compartment release relatively late may be subject to rhabdomyolysis and will require appropriate systemic treatment, in particular IV fluids and correction of electrolytes.[19]

Conclusion

Compartment syndrome remains a challenging condition but significant morbidity can be avoided by prompt diagnosis and decompression using a careful two-incision fasciotomy technique.

References

1. Pearse MF, Harry L, Nanchahal J. 2002: Acute compartment syndrome of the leg. Editorial. *BMJ*; **325**: 557–8.
2. Tiwari A, Haq AI, Myint F, Hamilton G. 2002: Acute compartment syndromes. *Br J Surg*; **89**: 397–412.
3. Janzing HM, Broos PL. 2001: Routine monitoring of compartment pressure in patients with tibial fractures: Beware of overtreatment! *Injury*; **32**: 415–21.
4. McQueen MM, Court-Brown CM. 1996: Compartment monitoring in tibial fractures. The pressure threshold for decompression. *J Bone Joint Surg Br*; **78**: 99–104.
5. Harris IA, Kadir A, Donald G. 2006: Continuous compartment pressure monitoring for tibia fractures: Does it influence outcome? *J Trauma*; **60**: 1330–5; discussion 1335.
6. Williams PR, Russell ID, Mintowt-Czyz WJ. 1998: Compartment pressure monitoring—current UK orthopaedic practice. *Injury*; **29**: 229–32.
7. Boody AR, Wongworawat MD. 2005: Accuracy in the measurement of compartment pressures: A comparison of three commonly used devices. *J Bone Joint Surg Am*; **87**: 2415–22.
8. Uliasz A, Ishida JT, Fleming JK, Yamamoto LG. 2003: Comparing the methods of measuring compartment pressures in acute compartment syndrome. *Am J Emerg Med*; **21**: 143–5.
9. Fitzgerald AM, Gaston P, Wilson Y, Quaba A, McQueen MM. 2000: Long-term sequelae of fasciotomy wounds. *Br J Plast Surg*; **53**: 690–3.
10. Cohen MS, Garfin SR, Hargens AR, Mubarak SJ. 1991: Acute compartment syndrome. Effect of dermotomy on fascial decompression in the leg. *J Bone Joint Surg Br*; **73**: 287–90.
11. Mubarak SJ, Owen CA. 1977: Double-incision fasciotomy of the leg for decompression in compartment syndromes. *J Bone Joint Surg Am*; **59**: 184–7.
12. British Orthopaedic Association/British Association of Plastic Surgeons. 1997: A report by the British Orthopaedic Association/British Association of Plastic Surgeons Working Party on the Management of Open Tibial Fractures. September 1997. *Br J Plast Surg*; **50**: 570–83.
13. Johnson SB, Weaver FA, Yellin AE, Kelly R, Bauer M. 1992: Clinical results of decompressive dermotomy-fasciotomy. *Am J Surg*; **164**: 286–90.
14. Bermudez K, Knudson MM, Morabito D, Kessel O. 1998: Fasciotomy, chronic venous insufficiency, and the calf muscle pump. *Arch Surg*; **133**: 1356–61.
15. Klenerman L. 2007: The evolution of the compartment syndrome since 1948 as recorded in the JBJS (B). *J Bone Joint Surg Br*; **89**: 1280–2.
16. Reis ND, Better OS. 2005: Mechanical muscle-crush injury and acute muscle-crush compartment syndrome: With special reference to earthquake casualties. *J Bone Joint Surg Br*; **87**: 450–3.
17. Finkelstein JA, Hunter GA, Hu RW. 1996: Lower limb compartment syndrome: Course after delayed fasciotomy. *J Trauma*; **40**: 342–4.
18. Vaillancourt C, Shrier I, Vandal A, *et al.* 2004 : Acute compartment syndrome: How long before muscle necrosis occurs? *CJEM*; **6**: 147–54.
19. Bagley WH, Yang H, Shah KH. 2007: Rhabdomyolysis. *Intern Emerg Med*; **2**: 210–8.

14 VASCULAR INJURIES

Principal recommendations

1. Devascularized limbs are a surgical emergency. They are recognized immediately and require urgent surgical exploration. The aim is to restore circulation within 3–4 h of the injury, after which muscle death begins. The maximum acceptable delay is 6 h of warm ischaemia time.
2. Capillary refill in the toes can be misleading and, if the circulation is not normal compared to the contralateral limb, there is a low threshold for exploration.
3. Absent peripheral pulses are not attributed to vascular spasm or compartment syndrome. A major vascular injury is always considered and senior surgical opinion is sought.
4. Preoperative angiography in the devascularized limb wastes valuable time. It is possible to define the level of injury from the fracture configuration and site of any dislocation.
5. Shunting significantly reduces the morbidity associated with these injuries by reducing the ischaemic time. Muscle suffers irreversible ischaemic damage within 3–4 h of complete ischaemia. Nerves are also susceptible to ischaemic injury.
6. Once the circulation is restored, the limb is reassessed with regards to the potential for salvage.
7. The skeleton is then stabilized before replacing the shunts with reversed vein grafts.
8. Proximal to the level of the trifurcation, any deep venous injury is also reconstructed.
9. Access incisions for vascular repair take into account the necessity for flap cover and the presence of adjacent fractures.
10. Fasciotomy is performed if indicated by the presence of raised intracompartmental pressures compared to the diastolic blood pressure. However, it is important that these measurements are performed repeatedly, as muscle swelling may not develop until several hours after revascularization (see Chapter 13).
11. The presence of a single patent artery to the foot is not a contraindication to free flap reconstruction using end-to-side anastomoses. In this situation, reconstruction of the injured vessels is considered, especially the posterior tibial artery.

Literature review

Devascularized limb

The most important factors in the treatment of the limb with vascular compromise are recognition that there is a significant vascular injury and re-establishing the circulation within 3–4 h of the injury.[1] Beyond this time, irreversible muscle damage will have occurred and revascularization may result in systemic problems, including myoglobinuria, renal failure and even death. Howard and Makin[2] found a correlation between delayed revascularization and amputation, with a 50% amputation rate in those revascularized after 8 h. These authors also suggested that preoperative angiography is unnecessary. Braten *et al*[3] reviewed 11 grade IIIC fractures and found that four of six patients with an ischaemic time of more than 8 h suffered massive muscle necrosis. Lange *et al*[4] also found that delay of more than 6 h was associated with worse outcome.

Devascularization appears to be more common with displaced fractures of the femur and posterior fracture dislocations of the knee than with fractures of the tibial shaft. Recognition of the injury requires a high index of suspicion.

Simple examination for capillary return in the toes can be misleading. Blood pooled in the extremity can be expressed on pressure and refills on release, giving the appearance of capillary refill. Palpation of the posterior tibial and dorsalis pedis pulses is recommended and, if this is not possible because of swelling, a Doppler ultrasound machine can be used. If the vessels are kinked, then reduction of the fracture may restore the circulation, provided the patient is systemically stable and has a good filling pressure. If in doubt, it is prudent to assume that the patient has a vascular injury. Waiting for angiography wastes valuable time.[1] It cannot be assumed that vascular compromise is due to an intimal tear, a thrombus, vascular spasm or compartment syndrome. Faris *et al*[5] reviewed 122 lower limb arterial injuries and found that only two had a tear or spasm and all required treatment with a reverse vein graft. The site of the vascular injury can be predicted from the fracture configuration.[2] An on-table angiogram can be performed by making an incision in the groin, locating the femoral artery and injecting contrast medium directly into it, with compression proximally.

Direct surgical exploration of the suspected site of vascular injury is recommended. Passing Fogarty catheters is unhelpful. These injuries do not behave like chronically ischaemic limbs in atherosclerotic patients. The incisions are placed so as not to compromise any reconstructive flap options. Once the site of injury has been identified, the limb can be immediately revascularized using vascular shunts,[1] e.g. carotid (Javid) shunts or Pruitt shunts. Placing the latter is easier, but they are of a smaller calibre. If the femoral or popliteal vein has also been injured, this should also be shunted. Locating the veins is easy once the arterial circulation has been established. It is vital to alert the anaesthetist once the limb has been reperfused because products from the ischaemic limb entering the systemic circulation often result in a drop in the blood pressure. A forced diuresis may be necessary for myoglobinuria and catheterization of the bladder to monitor urine output and quality is essential. Once the shunts are in place, the surgeon has time to reassess the patient and the limb. There is an extensive literature supporting the use of shunts.[6–11]

If the limb appears to be salvageable, the fracture can then be stabilized with an external fixator. McHenry et al[12] recommend revascularization before skeletal fixation, with a lower fasciotomy rate of 36% compared to 80% in those fixed first and hence delaying revascularization. It is important not to dislodge the shunts and hence stabilization with a simple bridging external fixator is preferred.

Definitive reconstruction of the vascular defect with vein grafts is preferred to prosthetic materials. The cephalic vein may be a better source of material than the saphenous vein as the wall is less muscular and prone to spasm, and it also readily dilates to accommodate the increased flow. It is preferable not to cross-clamp the vessels for insertion of vein grafts until the limb has been reperfused for at least 2 h. Ideally, the vein grafts, or at least the anastomoses, should be covered with local tissues but this can sometimes be difficult to achieve because of the swelling.

A systematic review of the literature identified 101 open fractures associated with devascularization of the lower limb.[1] The data confirmed that angiography causes unnecessary delays and that the optimal sequence of reconstruction to reduce warm ischaemia time and improve limb salvage is the insertion of vascular shunts, skeletal fixation followed by definitive vascular reconstruction using autologous vein grafts.

Venous repair

Proximal to the trifurcation, the veins should be reconstructed as well as the arteries. Kuralay et al[13] assessed the outcome of venous repair in 97 patients, 47 of whom had associated fractures. Proximal repairs had higher patency rates (common femoral 100%, superficial femoral 89%, popliteal 86%) at 1 year compared to all infrapopliteal repairs being thrombosed at 1 day post op.

Single vessel leg

Fracture of the fibula may disrupt the peroneal vessels as they lie in close proximity to the bone. Displaced fractures of the tibia, and especially ankle fracture dislocations, may injure the anterior tibial vessels. Thus, a leg and foot supplied by a single artery is not uncommon following these high energy injuries. It is important to recognize this situation as these fractures often require free tissue transfer for soft tissue reconstruction. There are no contraindications to using an end-to-side anastomosis for an isolated patent artery but this depends on an adequate rate of flow. Preoperative angiography is useful in providing a 'road map' but does not show the rate of flow or provide any information on the status of the venae commitans.

Segmental arterial injury

This should be suspected clinically from the zone of injury and only careful study of the angiograms will reveal the problem as a less well-filled segment of artery. It has important implications for arterial microsurgical anastomoses downstream, as flow may be severely compromised, predisposing to flap failure. This type of injury is especially important when the posterior tibial artery is involved and may not be accompanied by significant injury to the nerve.

Vascular injury and outcome

Revascularization should not be attempted simply because it is technically possible. The overall status of the patient should be considered and the option of below-knee amputation should be discussed.

The presence of vascular injuries appears to be predictive of the outcome in terms of fracture healing, infection and swelling. Dickson *et al*[14] studied 114 limbs by arteriography. Sixty-two had normal arteriograms whilst 52 had one or more vessels injured. Patients with grade IIIC injuries were excluded. The vascular injury group had an approximately three-fold higher rate of delayed or non-union and more infections. Waikakul *et al*[15] randomized Grade IIIA and IIIB fractures (IIIC fractures excluded) to vascular (arterial and venous) repair or not. Those in the vascular repair group had lower infection rate, more rapid fracture union, less chronic foot swelling and atrophic changes, as well as a reduced need for blood transfusion.

Conclusion

It is imperative that the devascularized limb is recognized and explored promptly. Preoperative angiography prolongs the ischaemic time unnecessarily. The use of shunts results in prompt revascularization. The fracture can then be stabilized before the insertion of reversed vein grafts.

References

1. Glass GE, Pearse MF, Nanchahal J. 2009: Improving lower limb salvage following fractures with vascular injury: A systematic review and new management algorithm. *J Plast Reconstr Aesthet Surg*; **62**: 571–9.
2. Howard PW, Makin GS. 1990: Lower limb fractures with associated vascular injury. *J Bone Joint Surg Br*; **72**: 116–20.
3. Braten M, Helland P, Myhre HO, Molster A, Terjesen T. 1996: 11 femoral fractures with vascular injury: Good outcome with early vascular repair and internal fixation. *Acta Orthop Scand*; **67**: 161–4.
4. Lange RH, Bach AW, Hansen ST Jr, Johansen KH. 1985: Open tibial fractures with associated vascular injuries: Prognosis for limb salvage. *J Trauma*; **25**: 203–8.
5. Faris IB, Raptis S, Fitridge R. 1997: Arterial injury in the lower limb from blunt trauma. *Aust N Z J Surg*; **67**: 25–30.

6. Johansen K, Bandyk D, Thiele B, Hansen ST Jr. 1982: Temporary intraluminal shunts: Resolution of a management dilemma in complex vascular injuries. *J Trauma*; **22**: 395–402.
7. Khalil IM, Livingston DH. 1986: Intravascular shunts in complex lower limb trauma. *J Vasc Surg*; **4**: 582–7.
8. Majeski JA, Gauto A. 1979: Management of peripheral arterial vascular injuries with a Javid shunt. *Am J Surg*; **138**: 324–5.
9. Nichols JG, Svoboda JA, Parks SN. 1986: Use of temporary intraluminal shunts in selected peripheral arterial injuries. *J Trauma*; **26**: 1094–6.
10. Reber PU, Patel AG, Sapio NL, Ris HB, Beck M, Kniemeyer HW. 1999: Selective use of temporary intravascular shunts in coincident vascular and orthopedic upper and lower limb trauma. *J Trauma*; **47**: 72–6.
11. Rozycki GS, Tremblay LN, Feliciano DV, McClelland WB. 2003: Blunt vascular trauma in the extremity: Diagnosis, management, and outcome. *J Trauma*; **55**: 814–24.
12. McHenry TP, Holcomb JB, Aoki N, Lindsey RW. 2002: Fractures with major vascular injuries from gunshot wounds: Implications of surgical sequence. *J Trauma*; **53**: 717–21.
13. Kuralay E, Demirkilic U, Ozal E, *et al.* 2002: A quantitative approach to lower extremity vein repair. *J Vasc Surg*; **36**: 1213–8.
14. Dickson K, Katzman S, Delgado E, Contreras D. 1994: Delayed unions and nonunions of open tibial fractures. Correlation with arteriography results. *Clin Orthop Relat Res*; **302**: 189–93.
15. Waikakul S, Sakkarnkosol S, Vanadurongwan V. 1998: Vascular injuries in compound fractures of the leg with initially adequate circulation. *J Bone Joint Surg Br*; **80**: 254–8.

15 OPEN FRACTURES OF THE FOOT AND ANKLE

Principal recommendations

1. These are particularly challenging injuries owing to the limited local soft tissue flap options, likelihood of injury to the neurovascular bundles, intra-articular fractures predisposing to poor long-term function and difficulty in stabilizing the fractures.
2. Amputation is considered when the final functional outcome following reconstruction is likely to be inferior to a transtibial amputation. This is especially likely to be the case for a 'floating ankle' injury or crush injuries with an open mid- and fore-foot.
3. Initial skeletal stabilization is achieved with a spanning external fixator, avoiding fibular plating. There are inherent difficulties in stabilizing these fractures as the anchor points for most spanning external fixators rely on an intact os calcis/talus/metatarsals.
4. Definitive skeletal fixation is performed at the time of soft tissue coverage. The exact configuration will depend on the fracture pattern, with intra-articular fractures usually best managed by internal fixation. Internal fixation is not recommended in the absence of adequate soft tissue cover as this may be associated with an increased risk of deep sepsis.
5. Degloved plantar skin:
    (a) If suprafascial, is defatted and replaced as full-thickness graft
    (b) If subfascial and proximally based, is sutured back without tension
    (c) If subfascial and distally based, is considered for revascularization.
6. Plantar soft tissue loss is best managed using fasciocutaneous flaps and reinnervation may confer some protection against the development of neuropathic ulceration. Dorsal skin loss can be managed by split skin grafts or thin, free fasciocutaneous flaps.
7. Open pilon fractures are stabilised with a spanning external fixator. If the planned definitive treatment is internal fixation of the tibial plafond, and provided the soft tissues permit, open reduction and internal fixation of the fibula at primary surgery may help to assist maintain the limb out to length. Soft tissue cover should be by way of thin, pliable fasciocutaneous flaps.
8. Injuries to the posterior tibial nerve are accurately assessed and consideration is given to reconstruction of segmental defects of the posterior tibial artery with autologous vascular graft. End-to-end anastomoses to avulsed vessels are performed with care as it can be difficult to assess the extent of intimal damage.

9. Open hind-foot injuries are managed as for a diaphyseal injury when only one articular surface is involved. When there is greater disruption of the hind-foot, a transtibial amputation is considered.
10. Isolated open mid-foot injuries are often caused by heavy objects falling on the foot. These result in significant postoperative stiffness and pain due to ligamentous disruption and again, amputation is considered.
11. Open fore-foot injuries involving the first metatarsal are treated as aggressively as open diaphyseal injuries. When the other metatarsals are injured in isolation, a ray amputation results in a reasonable return to ambulation.

Literature review

Salvage or amputate?

The significance of high-energy open foot and ankle injuries is the threat of amputation.

The foot is the 'end organ' of the lower limb and can, if ill-advised attempts at salvage are made, hinder walking to a greater extent than prosthetic replacement. There are no absolute indications for amputation and the decision threshold is altered based on the overall injury, anticipated function after reconstruction, concomitant injuries particularly if life threatening, and the facilities and resources available to offer salvage. The following scenarios should prompt consideration of amputation over salvage and reconstruction:

1. A 'floating' open ankle injury – severe open distal tibial and hind-foot fractures
2. Open mid- and fore-foot injuries sustained through crushing, which often lead to severe stiffness and pain.

Management of the skeletal injuries

A spanning external fixator is recommended in the first instance. A provisional reduction maintains length and facilitates better interpretation of subsequent imaging studies. Fibular plating is not necessary at index surgery if the limb is stabilized by external fixation. An isolated medial malleolar fracture, if reduced by closed means or through percutaneous manipulation, can be fixed by a single screw at the initial surgery.[1] Any further attempts at definitive reduction or fixation should be avoided at this stage.

Purchase of external fixator pins into the metatarsals (in extensive foot and ankle injuries), can still be supported by modern fixators, which allow 'suspension' of the extremity.

Definitive fixation will depend on fracture characteristics and the nature of soft tissue cover. In general, articular injuries are better held with internal fixation techniques. Unsalvageable joints can be fused using either internal or external fixation methods.

Specific injury patterns

The following are some of the injury patterns that may be encountered:

1. Plantar soft tissue injuries
2. Open injuries about the distal tibia involving the ankle joint
3. Open injuries of the talus and calcaneum
4. Open injuries of the mid-foot
5. Open injuries of the metatarsals

Plantar soft tissue injuries

Reconstruction of the plantar surface of the foot is possible. Sommerlad and Mc-Grouther[2] suggested that patients had a better gait when muscle flaps covered with split thickness skin grafts were used. However, extensive loss of the weight-bearing tissues over the heel and the lateral part of the foot and fore-foot can impose significant difficulty in fitting appropriate footwear for the prevention of neuropathic ulceration. In this scenario, a transtibial amputation is a viable alternative.[3] Recent publications[4] suggest thin fasciocutaneous flaps are superior, as they are less prone to ulceration and the innervation of these flaps may confer some protection against trophic ulceration. A novel variant is to apply the degloved plantar skin as a graft to the flap donor site and subsequently transfer the prefabricated flap to achieve plantar skin coverage on the weight-bearing surface of the foot.

Plantar degloving

Jeng and Wei[4] described treatment based on the pathoanatomy of the degloved skin. Tissues degloved in the suprafascial plane should be defatted and replaced as full-thickness skin grafts. Proximally-based subfascial degloved tissues should be sutured back without tension and, if distally based, microvascular revascularization should be considered. If the degloved tissue is not salvageable, their preferred option for reconstruction was with pedicled or free fasciocutaneous flaps.

Dorsal foot skin loss

These defects can be managed with skin grafts if the wound bed is suitable or, thin free fasciocutaneous flaps if required.[5]

Open injuries about the distal tibia involving the ankle joint

Soft tissues

Anterior soft tissue defects resulting from direct injury or hyperflexion of the ankle are often associated with avulsion of the anterior tibial vessels and, occasionally, disruption of the tendons. Reconstruction of the tibialis anterior and extensor hallucis longus tendons with grafts is recommended. Substantial loss of the extensor tendons of the lesser toes can be treated with interposition grafts or by tenodesis to the extensor retinaculum or adjacent fascial structures. Bowstringing of the tendons can be corrected by reconstruction of the extensor retinaculum. Soft tissue coverage should be achieved with thin fasciocutaneous flaps to avoid subsequent problems with footwear and to achieve the best cosmetic result.

Medial-sided soft tissue defects are associated with open distal tibial fractures. Lacerations and skin defects are usually transverse or oblique. Fractures lines may extend into the ankle joint. The medial thrust to the distal tibia, which pushes it out of the soft tissue envelope, also risks potential damage to the posterior tibial vessels. It is important to assess the zone of injury as traction can result in intimal damage and anastomoses should be performed proximal to this zone. If there is no flow through the posterior tibial artery and there is a suitable distal segment, consideration should be given to reconstruction of the damaged segment with autologous reversed vein graft. If necessary, free flaps can be anastomosed end to side to the graft. In general, the posterior tibial vessels are preferred to the anterior tibial vessels as recipients for free flaps.[6] The posterior tibial nerve may also suffer a traction injury but is rarely divided following blunt trauma. It is important to evaluate the plantar sensation before surgery and to inspect the external appearance of the nerve at the time of wound debridement for telltale signs of axonotmesis. Again, thin fasciocutaneous flaps are the preferred choice for reconstruction.

Skeletal injury

Timing of definitive fixation is as important in open injuries as in severe closed types. Initial spanning external fixation provides several advantages:

1. Stability to facilitate soft tissue recovery
2. Holding the skeletal tissues out to length and in approximate alignment, to enable better interpretation of subsequent imaging studies
3. Access for soft tissue surgery.

Distal tibial injuries can be managed definitively by external fixation (with or without minimal internal fixation to hold articular fragments) or by internal fixation using plates and screws.[7–10] Modern low-profile contoured plates are available for anterior, medial, lateral and posterior surfaces of the tibia. Use of these implants ideally should coincide with definitive soft tissue cover. Even so, deep infection rates of 10% are reported with the higher grade of open injuries,[11] especially with medial-sided implants.

Involvement of the foot as well as the distal tibia produces a 'floating ankle.' This term is borrowed from 'floating knee,' when concurrent femoral and tibial fractures give rise to a joint bereft of anatomical continuity with the remainder of the appendicular skeleton. It is a pattern of injury that requires close coordination of orthoplastic surgical efforts. Reconstruction is often a staged process and amputation is a viable alternative.[12,13] Definitive fixation will depend on the fracture patterns and quality of soft tissue cover. Internal fixation of articular fractures in the presence of a clean wound and with provision of simultaneous soft tissue cover is preferred. Otherwise, external fixation is recommended. It may also be possible to combine both techniques.[1,12,13]

The complexity of these injuries warrants treatment by specialists who are not only experts in their surgical disciplines but collaborate regularly across the orthoplastic spectrum. Prompt referral to these centres is recommended. Attempts to treat these injuries definitively at non-specialist centres is discouraged as the initial surgical efforts may need to be taken down before reconstruction is possible.[1] Provisional stabilization through spanning external fixation is the optimum method of 'damage control' prior to transfer.

Open injuries of the talus and calcaneum
Soft tissue

Soft tissue loss over the calcaneum poses a difficult challenge. Localized areas of soft tissue loss over the heel ideally are treated by local, innervated flaps, and the medial islanded plantar instep flap is ideal. More extensive defects require distant or free thin fasciocutaneous flaps and there is some evidence to suggest that reinnervated flaps may confer some benefit.[14,15]

Skeletal injury

The talus and calcaneum are part of four major joints (ankle, subtalar, calcaneocuboid and calcaneonavicular). Disruption of any of these can lead to significant compromise in hind- and mid-foot function. Whilst there is controversy regarding the treatment of closed calcaneal fractures,[16] the issues in open injuries are different. Surgery is essential for wound excision, stabilization and cover. Successful management of open talar and calcaneal injuries is a formidable challenge.[17] Acute management is according to guidelines in this publication: assessment by orthopaedic and plastic surgeons, debridement and provisional stabilization. In the event of joint dislocations (ankle or subtalar), these are reduced at primary surgery. Temporary stabilization by Kirschner wires will augment the spanning external fixator. The extruded talus is an extreme variant of fracture dislocation; published series are small owing to the rare nature of the event.[18,19] Definitive guidelines are lacking and the decision to reimplant should be made on the presence of other associated injuries, degree of contamination of the talus and state of the extruded bone (articular cartilage damage, fractures within the talus). Reimplantation can be associated with a high infection rate and subsequent necessity for talectomy and tibiocalcaneal arthrodesis.

Reduction and definitive fixation of talar neck and body fractures should also be performed at the time of primary surgery if possible. This is to reduce potential development of osteonecrosis of the talus, perhaps through preservation of whatever tenuous blood supply remains.

The majority (93%) of open calcaneal fractures have a medial soft tissue defect with a significant proportion (25%) sustaining posterior tibial neurovascular injury.[17] Fracture patterns are often complex and not fully appreciated until better imaging is obtained. High deep infection rates have been reported with internal fixation,[20] although current strategies to perform 'interval' fixation, i.e. after soft tissue conditions have been fully declared and managed, appear to reduce the complication rate.[21–23] Definitive soft tissue cover should accompany internal fixation. If the two procedures cannot be undertaken simultaneously, then the soft tissues take priority. Alternatives to plate and screw fixation include circular external fixators or mini-external fixators used within the confines of a spanning external fixator.[24–26] Salvage can be successful as long as deep sepsis is avoided – management of the skeletal injury must not compromise that of soft tissues.[20]

Open injuries of the mid-foot

The mid-foot spans the area between the talus and calcaneum proximally and the metatarsal bases distally. The integument of this part of the foot (like the ankle) is thin and easily injured. In a review of crush injuries to the mid-foot by Chandran *et al*,[27] in which the majority were managed through a combination of external fixation and split thickness skin grafts, almost all exhibited severe morbidity (stiffness and pain) 1 year after fixator removal. The complexity of the mid-foot as a structural and functional link between hind- and fore-foot should not be underestimated and an amputation should be considered in severe injuries where reconstruction potentially yields a stiff painful foot.

Open injuries of the metatarsals

A solitary open metatarsal fracture is treated in line with the general guidelines. Multiple fractures often occur in association with crush injuries and management of the soft tissue envelope takes priority. Management of dorsal skin loss has been described above. Spanning external fixation is appropriate in the acute phase. The absence of suitable fixation points for half pins in the metatarsals necessitates the use of fixation points in the tibia and os calcis to construct a frame which elevates the entire foot off the bed. In a report of 10 patients with open metatarsal fractures, four Gustilo grade IIIB injuries subsequently required ray amputations.[28] The published data highlight the severity of these injuries.

References

1. Khan U, Smitham P, Pearse M, Nanchahal J. 2007: Management of severe open ankle injuries. *Plast Reconstr Surg*; **119**: 578–89.
2. Sommerlad BC, McGrouther DA. 1978: Resurfacing the sole: Long-term follow-up and comparison of techniques. *Br J Plast Surg*; **31**: 107–16.
3. Uroskie T, Colen L. 2001: Soft tissue reconstruction for the heel and plantar foot. *Foot Ankle Clin*; **6**: 801–26.

4. Jeng SF, Wei FC. 1997: Classification and reconstructive options in foot plantar skin avulsion injuries. *Plast Reconstr Surg*; **99**: 1695–703; discussion 1704–5.
5. Yang WG, Chiang YC, Wei FC, Feng GM, Chen KT. 2006: Thin anterolateral thigh perforator flap using a modified perforator microdissection technique and its clinical application for foot resurfacing. *Plast Reconstr Surg*; **117**: 1004–8.
6. Chen HC, Chuang CC, Chen S, Hsu WM, Wei FC. 1994: Selection of recipient vessels for free flaps to the distal leg and foot following trauma. *Microsurgery*; **15**: 358–63.
7. Leung F, Kwok HY, Pun TS, Chow SP. 2004: Limited open reduction and Ilizarov external fixation in the treatment of distal tibial fractures. *Injury*; **35**: 278–83.
8. Bacon S, Smith WR, Morgan SJ, *et al.* 2008: A retrospective analysis of comminuted intra-articular fractures of the tibial plafond: Open reduction and internal fixation versus external Ilizarov fixation. *Injury*; **39**: 196–202.
9. Wyrsch B, McFerran MA, McAndrew M, *et al.* 1996: Operative treatment of fractures of the tibial plafond. A randomized, prospective study. *J Bone Joint Surg Am*; **78**: 1646–57.
10. Marsh JL, Borrelli J Jr, Dirschl DR, Sirkin MS. 2007: Fractures of the tibial plafond. *Instr Course Lect*; **56**: 331–52.
11. Sirkin M, Sanders R, DiPasquale T, Herscovici D Jr. 2004: A staged protocol for soft tissue management in the treatment of complex pilon fractures. *J Orthop Trauma*; **18** (Suppl): S32–8.
12. Debnath UK, Maripuri SN, Guha AR, Parfitt D, Fournier C, Hariharan K. 2007: Open grade III "floating ankle" injuries: A report of eight cases with review of literature. *Arch Orthop Trauma Surg*; **127**: 625–31.
13. McHale KA, Gajewski DA. 2002: The "floating ankle": A pattern of violent injury. Treatment with thin-pin external fixation. *Mil Med*; **167**: 454–8.
14. Koski EA, Kuokkanen HO, Koskinen SK, Tukiainen EJ. 2004: Reconstruction of soft tissue after complicated calcaneal fractures. *Scand J Plast Reconstr Surg Hand Surg*; **38**: 284–7.
15. Attinger C, Cooper P. 2001: Soft tissue reconstruction for calcaneal fractures or osteomyelitis. *Orthop Clin North Am*; **32**: 135–70.
16. Bajammal S, Tornetta P 3rd, Sanders D, Bhandari M. 2005: Displaced intra-articular calcaneal fractures. *J Orthop Trauma*; **19**: 360–4.
17. Lawrence SJ, Singhal M. 2007: Open hindfoot injuries. *J Am Acad Orthop Surg*; **15**: 367–76.
18. Detenbeck LC, Kelly PJ. 1969: Total dislocation of the talus. *J Bone Joint Surg Am*; **51**: 283–8.
19. Assal M, Stern R. 2004: Total extrusion of the talus. A case report. *J Bone Joint Surg Am*; **86**: 2726–31.
20. Siebert CH, Hansen M, Wolter D. 1998: Follow-up evaluation of open intra-articular fractures of the calcaneus. *Arch Orthop Trauma Surg*; **117**: 442–7.
21. Berry GK, Stevens DG, Kreder HJ, McKee M, Schemitsch E, Stephen DJ. 2004: Open fractures of the calcaneus: A review of treatment and outcome. *J Orthop Trauma*; **18**: 202–6.
22. Benirschke SK, Kramer PA. 2004: Wound healing complications in closed and open calcaneal fractures. *J Orthop Trauma*; **18**: 1–6.
23. Aldridge JM 3rd, Easley M, Nunley JA. 2004: Open calcaneal fractures: results of operative treatment. *J Orthop Trauma*; **18**: 7–11.
24. Emara KM, Allam MF. 2005: Management of calcaneal fracture using the Ilizarov technique. *Clin Orthop Relat Res*; **439**: 215–20.
25. McGarvey WC, Burris MW, Clanton TO, Melissinos EG. 2006: Calcaneal fractures: indirect reduction and external fixation. *Foot Ankle Int*; **27**: 494–9.
26. Magnan B, Bortolazzi R, Marangon A, Marino M, Dall'Oca C, Bartolozzi P. 2006: External fixation for displaced intra-articular fractures of the calcaneum. *J Bone Joint Surg Br*; **88**: 1474–9.
27. Chandran P, Puttaswamaiah R, Dhillon MS, Gill SS. 2006: Management of complex open fracture injuries of the midfoot with external fixation. *J Foot Ankle Surg*; **45**: 308–15.
28. Hoxie S, Turner NS, 3rd, Strickland J, Jacofsky D. 2007: Clinical course of open metatarsal fractures. *Orthopedics*; **30**: 662–5.

16 WHEN THINGS GO WRONG WITH SOFT TISSUES

Principal recommendations

1. Necrosis of a local flap over the fracture site is managed by early return to theatre and revision surgery to achieve healthy soft tissue coverage.
2. Limited tip congestion may respond to leech therapy.
3. Some local fasciocutaneous flaps may be more prone to develop complications in patients with comorbidities.
4. Free flap complications are reduced by patient preparation, careful planning and performing the anastomoses outside the zone of injury: ideally proximally.
5. There is a low threshold for immediate re-exploration of a free flap with suspected circulatory compromise.
6. Deep infection requires a return to the operating theatre, fracture site exploration, debridement, dead space management and antibiotic therapy. Fracture fixation may need revision.

Flap loss

Flap loss can be minor in the form of zonal necrosis, e.g. tip necrosis in local fasciocutaneous flaps, or total necrosis. These complications must be approached in an individual manner. However, there are some principles which may help in ensuring optimal outcome.

Local flaps

Tip necrosis of a local flap

The tip of a fasciocutaneous flap is usually the least well-vascularized part and is most vulnerable to this complication. Tip necrosis, whilst always unwelcome, may only be a nuisance in other areas. However, for open fractures it is usually the region over or immediately adjacent to the fracture that is affected. Whilst surgeon-dependent factors such as poor flap selection, design or execution may render the flap more prone to this complication, patients with comorbidities such as diabetes, peripheral vascular disease and older age may be more susceptible to this problem.[1] Tip necrosis can affect as many as 10% of cases.[2] Use of rheological agents such as low molecular weight dextran may help but should be used with care in the elderly as there is a real risk of cardiovascular complications.[3] The use of topical vasodilatory agents is of limited benefit.[4]

Once tip necrosis has declared itself (usually within 72 h of showing initial signs of vascular compromise), the patient must be returned to theatre for revision surgery. Obviously, in the presence of infection, surgery should not be delayed. Occasionally, it is possible to excise the necrotic tip, advance the flap and reinset it. If this is not possible, the surgeon may have to consider alternative flap coverage, including free tissue transfer.

Total necrosis of a local flap

There may be doubt with respect to the viability of the entire flap when it is first elevated. This concern should be addressed immediately with a change in surgical strategy. The flap may be returned as a delay procedure or the surgeon may consider alternative flap coverage, such as using a free flap.

Delayed compromise of the entire local flap often is due to venous congestion. The venae commitans of the distally-based fasciocutaneous flaps have a variable anatomical relationship to the perforating arteries.[5] When islanding these distal flaps, attention should be given to securing the best configuration for the draining veins after flap inset. The early management of venous congestion is to ensure that extrinsic factors such as haematoma or tight dressings are not responsible for compression of the draining veins. Once this has been addressed, decompression of the intrinsic circulation to salvage the flap should be undertaken. Use of medicinal leeches[6,7] and rheological agents is a recognized method to achieve decompression and assist intrinsic circulation. Antibiotic prophylaxis using a fluroquinolone to cover against *Aeromonas* infection from the leeches must be instigated as more than one-third of patients may develop infection.[8]

Free flaps

In a 10-year retrospective review of free tissue transfer in lower limb reconstruction, Wettstein *et al*[9] reported a 40% complication rate ranging from wound dehiscence to total flap loss, with patient age identified as the only factor associated with increased flap loss. Free flaps can suffer from zonal necrosis if the choke vessels to the respective angiosome are insufficient or if sufficient perforators are not included in the pedicle. This is a particular problem if the fracture underlies the non-viable section of the flap.

Early anastomotic failure

Careful technique should address immediate technical issues, such as narrowing the lumen of the anastomosis by inadvertently picking up the back wall with a suture.

Intrinsic causes of anastomotic failure often present within 1 h of clamp removal.[10] Thus, a defensive approach would be to allow this period of time to elapse prior to moving the patient out of theatre or the recovery area. If after repeat anastomosis, the vessels fail to run, then a change in surgical strategy is recommended.

The problems may be either on the flap or recipient side and a decision must be made as to which is most likely. Perhaps the simplest technique for evaluating the arterial outflow is by removing the clamp from the recipient artery and assessing the arterial outflow ('spurt test'). A similar procedure can be performed for the recipient veins to assess back flow but this can be misleading as the back flow may be curtailed by the presence of valves. If the problems lie on the flap side (intimal damage through traction or poor flap design), then a second free flap may be considered.[11] The choice of second free flap should be based on those which are relatively easy to harvest and have a predictable vascular supply.

Recipient vessel problems can be arterial or venous, or both. If arterial and the problem is thought to be related to technical factors, then conversion of an end-to-side anastomosis to an end-to-end one may be considered. If the problem relates to the zone of injury, then a more proximal anastomosis, perhaps using a vein graft, should be considered.[12] Anastomosing to another axial vessel should be avoided for fear of devascularizing the foot. Recipient venous problems relate either to technical issues, often due to size discrepancy, or a proximal thrombus. If available, the superficial veins should be used when the deep veins are of small calibre or contain a thrombus. If the superficial veins are also not suitable, then a vein graft should be considered. Occasionally, thrombectomy by gently milking out the clot is successful.

If veins grafts do not permit straddling of an extensive zone of injury, then very rarely a cross-leg free flap may be considered, utilizing the uninjured vessels of the contralateral limb as recipient vessels.[13] Both limbs must be immobilized to prevent inadvertent movement and avulsion at the site of anastomoses, and this is most easily achieved using an external fixator.

It is essential that the patient only leaves the operating theatre when the senior operating surgeon is absolutely certain that the free flap is running well. Finally, if all reasonable attempts have failed, it is probably better to remove the unsuccessful flap, cover the fracture with a dressing and return on another day once the patient has been optimized, investigated and consented for further procedures, perhaps with the assistance of another team, rather than persist with further attempts late into the day, when the surgical, nursing and anaesthetic teams are tiring. Futile further attempts run the risk of making the situation worse.

Delayed anastomotic failure

The chances of successfully salvaging the flap depend upon the time delay between the development of flap embarrassment and restoration of flap circulation.[14] In order to reduce this time interval, reliable methods of flap monitoring by experienced staff must be in place. Ideally, the flap should be monitored continuously or at short, regular intervals. There is considerable variation in flap monitoring protocols.[15,16] The majority (90%) of arterial thromboses occur within the first 24 h, whilst 41% of venous failures occur after this time.[17] Venous anastomotic problems are almost three times commoner than arterial,[17] although clinical signs of venous congestion as manifest by swelling and colour changes may not be apparent for some time. Adjunctive techniques such as laser Doppler flow can detect changes in flap perfusion 1–3 h before clinical changes are apparent to experienced staff[18] and, when combined with strict protocols[19] or with tissue spectrophotometry,[20] the false-negative and -positive rates can be reduced.

Once flap compromise has been identified, it is imperative that the patient is returned to the operating theatre as soon as possible.[21] Half-hearted measures on the ward, such as releasing sutures for haematoma, simply waste valuable time. Once in theatre, both venous and arterial anastomoses are inspected critically. Any thrombus is gently removed and the flap circulation re-established. If the thrombosis extends into the microcirculation, streptokinase (50 000-250 000 units administered as 5000 units/ml) may be delivered directly into the artery of the flap and, following clamping of the outflow for approximately 20 min, the vein is disconnected to allow outflow of the thrombolytic agent to avoid systemic complications. After successful salvage, systemic anticoagulation with heparin should be considered.[22]

Other 'minor' complications

Loss of skin graft can lead to bacterial colonization. Return to theatre for this and other complications, such as a dehisced donor site, may be deferred for the first 3–5 days to avoid possible free flap anastomotic problems due to hypothermia or hypotension.

Slow healing of skin graft donor sites can be avoided by optimizing general patient factors such as nutrition, as well as considering elective over-grafting using widely meshed grafts in the elderly and appropriate management of dressings.

Cellulitis or other forms of superficial infection affecting the soft tissues should be managed aggressively by microbial cultures and immediate high dose antibiotic therapy.

Deep infection

In a recent retrospective review from a trauma centre, one-third of patients suffered from soft tissue infections and one-quarter from deep infections.[23] Deep infection, manifest once successful soft tissue coverage has been achieved, usually is related to the underlying fracture and necessitates close coordination between the plastic and orthopaedic surgical teams. The flap will need to be elevated and the problem treated by removal of any deep metalwork as appropriate, collection of deep specimens for microbiology and histology, and appropriate excision of bone and soft tissue (see Chapters 5 and 6). The only means of overcoming this challenging problem is to aim to convert the condition of the wound to that expected after the initial wound excision. The area of bone loss may then be treated with an antibiotic bead pouch (see Chapter 9) in preparation for reconstruction.

Soft tissue necrosis

Occasionally, the surgeon may be confronted with extensive soft tissue necrosis. Perhaps the commonest scenario is when a patient with established compartment syndrome undergoes late fasciotomy (see Chapter 13) and the necrotic muscle is exposed. In these instances, all the non-viable muscle should be resected and this often involves the entire compartment. Once the area has been adequately excised, the decision has to be made whether the limb can be salvaged by either direct closure of the skin or flap coverage or whether the patient would be best served by an amputation.[24] Whilst transtibial amputation can lead to a satisfactory final outcome, the function following through knee or transfemoral amputation is less satisfactory (see Chapter 18).

References

1. Baumeister SP, Spierer R, Erdmann D, Sweiss R, Levin LS, Germann GK. 2003: A realistic complication analysis of 70 sural artery flap in a multimorbid patient group. *Plast Reconstr Surg*; **112**: 129–40.
2. Erdmann MW, Court-Brown CM, Quaba AA. 1997: A five year review of islanded distally based fasciocutaneous flaps on the lower limb. *Br J Plast Surg*; **50**: 421–7.
3. Disa JJ, Polvora VP, Pusic AL, Singh B, Cordeiro PG. 2003: Dextran-related complications in head and neck microsurgery: do the benefits outweigh the risks? A prospective randomized analysis. *Plast Reconstr Surg*; **112**: 1534–9.
4. Uhl E, Rosken F, Curri SB, Menger MD, Messmer K. 1998: Reduction of skin flap necrosis by transdermal application of buflomedil bound to liposomes. *Plast Reconstr Surg*; **102**: 1598–604.
5. Ghali S, Bowman N, Khan U. 2005: The distal medial perforators of the lower leg and their accompanying veins. *Br J Plast Surg*; **58**: 1086–9.
6. Dabb RW, Malone JM, Leverett LC. 1992: The use of medicinal leeches in the salvage of flaps with venous congestion. *Ann Plast Surg*; **29**: 250-6.
7. Chepeha DB, Nussenbaum B, Bradford CR, Teknos TN. 2002: Leech therapy for patients with surgically unsalvageable venous obstruction after revascularized free tissue transfer. *Arch Otolaryngol Head Neck Surg*; **128**: 960–5.
8. Bauters TG, Buyle FM, Verschraegen G, *et al.* 2007: Infection risk related to the use of medicinal leeches. *Pharm World Sci*; **29**: 122–5.
9. Wettstein R, Schurch R, Banic A, Erni D, Harder Y. 2008: Review of 197 consecutive free flap reconstructions in the lower extremity. *J Plast Reconstr Aesthet Surg*; **61**: 772–6.
10. Wolff KD, Holzle F, Wysluch A, Mucke T, Kesting M. 2008: Incidence and time of intraoperative vascular complications in head and neck microsurgery. *Microsurgery*; **28**: 143–6.
11. Wei FC, Demirkan F, Chen HC, *et al.* 2001: The outcome of failed free flaps in head and neck and extremity reconstruction: what is next in the reconstructive ladder? *Plast Reconstr Surg*; **108**: 1154–60; discussion 1161–2.

12. Bayramicli M, Tetik C, Sonmez A, Gurunluoglu R, Baltaci F. 2002: Reliability of primary vein grafts in lower extremity free tissue transfers. *Ann Plast Surg*; **48**: 21–9.
13. Townsend PL. 1987: Indications and long-term assessment of 10 cases of cross-leg free DCIA flaps. *Ann Plast Surg*; **19**: 225–33.
14. Chen KT, Mardini S, Chuang DC, *et al.* 2007: Timing of presentation of the first signs of vascular compromise dictates the salvage outcome of free flap transfers. *Plast Reconstr Surg*; **120**: 187–95.
15. Whitaker IS, Oliver DW, Ganchi PA. 2003: Postoperative monitoring of microvascular tissue transfers: Current practice in the United Kingdom and Ireland. *Plast Reconstr Surg*; **111**: 2118–9.
16. Jallali N, Ridha H, Butler PE. 2005: Postoperative monitoring of free flaps in UK plastic surgery units. *Microsurgery*; **25**: 469–72.
17. Kroll SS, Schusterman MA, Reece GP, *et al.* 1996: Timing of pedicle thrombosis and flap loss after free-tissue transfer. *Plast Reconstr Surg*; **98**: 1230–3.
18. Clinton MS, Sepka RS, Bristol D, *et al.* 1991: Establishment of normal ranges of laser Doppler blood flow in autologous tissue transplants. *Plast Reconstr Surg*; **87**: 299–309.
19. Yuen JC, Feng Z. 2000: Monitoring free flaps using the laser Doppler flowmeter: Five-year experience. *Plast Reconstr Surg*; **105**: 55–61.
20. Holzle F, Loeffelbein DJ, Nolte D, Wolff KD. 2006: Free flap monitoring using simultaneous non-invasive laser Doppler flowmetry and tissue spectrophotometry. *J Craniomaxillofac Surg*; **34**: 25–33.
21. Hidalgo DA, Jones CS. 1990: The role of emergent exploration in free-tissue transfer: A review of 150 consecutive cases. *Plast Reconstr Surg*; **86**: 492–8; discussion 499–501.
22. Bui DT, Cordeiro PG, Hu QY, Disa JJ, Pusic A, Mehrara BJ. 2007: Free flap reexploration: Indications, treatment, and outcomes in 1193 free flaps. *Plast Reconstr Surg*; **119**: 2092–100.
23. Lo CH, Leung M, Baillieu C, Chong EW, Cleland H. 2007: Trauma centre experience: Flap reconstruction of traumatic lower limb injuries. *ANZ J Surg*; **77**: 690–4.
24. Finkelstein JA, Hunter GA, Hu RW. 1996: Lower limb compartment syndrome: Course after delayed fasciotomy. *J Trauma*; **40**: 342–4.

17 WHEN THINGS GO WRONG WITH BONE

1. Early complications with bone occur as a consequence of the original injury or from surgery.
2. Problems that present are:
   (a) Wound leakage
   (b) Sepsis
   (c) Loss of alignment.
3. Common causes include inadequate debridement, haematoma formation, inappropriate or delayed soft tissue cover and unstable fixation. Each cause is sought and remedied promptly.
4. An expectant approach is seldom fruitful and, if adopted, should be for a limited period only.
5. A decision to intervene is taken if there is failure to improve.
6. Early problems can exert an undue influence on the final outcome unless weighed for significance and acted upon appropriately and promptly.
7. Discussion of the case with the nearest specialist centre is encouraged and gives the opportunity to correct the problem at the earliest opportunity.

Problems associated with bone

The commonest early problems related to bony issues are wound leakage, sepsis and loss of alignment.

Wound leakage

This is unsuccessful primary healing of the soft tissue cover. Haematoma formation as a result of failure to eliminate 'dead space' at the time of wound cover is a major cause and can be confirmed by ultrasonography. The size and extent of the collection will determine if surgical evacuation is necessary. If localized and limited in size, an expectant approach with antibiotic cover is prudent. Failure of resolution within a few days should prompt surgical exploration. Haematoma under a flap may lead to flap necrosis.

Early sepsis

This is usually a consequence of inadequate debridement or delayed soft tissue cover. Strong published clinical evidence is lacking in terms of clear guidelines for the management of early infection after fracture stabilization. Some attempt is made in the literature to distinguish superficial from deep infection, but this is highly subjective. An infection of a skin grafted area may correctly be classed 'superficial', but all fracture and surgical wound infections are likely to represent a deep-seated problem. Suppression of infection by antibiotics until fracture union is often practised. This may be successful but a substantial proportion of patients will continue with symptoms requiring further surgery even after fracture union or implant removal. The approach to suppress early infection by antibiotics may best be reserved for less virulent pathogens, e.g. coagulase-negative staphylococcus. Gram-negative and meticillin-resistant *Staphylococcus aureus* infections are probably best treated by a revision of the surgical strategy.

In some cases, early infections may be overcome by prompt action. For example, when an intramedullary nail is used and problems occur at the fracture site, locking bolt wounds and (most worryingly of all) the nail entry point, this may herald the development of an intramedullary infection. Rising inflammatory markers (C-reactive protein) may provide an early warning. Early recognition and prompt treatment by exchange nailing with appropriate antibiotic cover may yield a rapid response.[1] However, if the infection is established, associated with a purulent discharge and caused by virulent bacteria, then implant removal, fracture site re-exploration with possible further debridement and resection, canal reaming and lavage may be necessary, and an external fixator used as the interim stabilization device. Then a decision can be made on how to deal with the problem definitively. Here an apparently successful initial treatment spirals into a true limb salvage scenario.

If internal fixation is introduced without the facility to provide immediate soft tissue cover, there is a rising incidence of infection proportional to the delay to wound closure.[2] This scenario is the equivalent of introducing any implant (e.g. an arthroplasty) and leaving the wound to be closed 24 or 48 h later. Most arthroplasty surgeons would not allow this to occur. The temptation to internally fix an open tibial fracture and 'leave closure to later by plastic surgery' is strongly discouraged.

Early sepsis may also be related to external fixator pins. Attention to pin placement outside the zone of injury is important. External fixator pin sites may become infected and, if placed within the zone of injury, the pin site (be it a threaded half pin or fine wire) will lie within tissue already compromised by the injury. Rapid propagation of the local infection may occur with possible skin necrosis and the potential to involve the fracture itself. A repositioning of the pin is needed.

Loss of alignment

If loss of alignment occurs early, it usually means the method for fracture stabilization was unsuitable rather than surgery inexpertly performed. The choice of fracture stabilization is, more often than not, made on surgeon familiarity and preference for a particular technique rather than suitability to the limb injury or fracture pattern. If malalignment is seen after primary stabilization, the question that needs to be considered is, was this the most suitable choice for this fracture pattern? If the answer is no, then revision is needed.

Internal fixation

The advantage of internal fixation is that it is a well-practised method of fracture fixation for most surgeons. Additionally, it is able to achieve good stability with most fracture patterns and provides easy access for plastic surgical reconstruction. However, reports of 'extended' indications for the use of certain methods of internal fixation – typically very distal and proximal tibial fractures treated by intramedullary nailing – require the incorporation of a modified technique not practised by most surgeons. Valgus and external rotation malalignment are common errors. Careful reduction and the use of interference (Poller) screws to steer the guide wire, reamers and nail in the correct path are needed.[3] These screws provide additional stability, without which hinging or toggling of the metaphyseal fragment will occur. A surgeon unfamiliar with the correct technique should opt for alternative means of stable fracture fixation.

External fixation

Poorly-sited external fixator pins fail if they are not configured appropriately. Pins connected to rods haphazardly (without attention to creating a 'module' on each side of the fracture and then connecting these to each other) can allow fragments to rotate on pins, causing pain and leading to loosening and loss of alignment. Another common cause of failure of external fixation is unsecured tightening of the various connections between pins, clamps and rods.

Well conceived and executed initial surgery will usually avoid these problems.[4] However, if there is any doubt about progress in wound healing, worsening pain, or the stability of the fracture fixation construct, then a thorough re-evaluation of the approach is essential. Early discussion with and referral to surgeons at the nearest specialist centre can avoid a protracted and uncertain attempt to salvage a difficult problem alone.

References

1. Court-Brown CM, Keating JF, McQueen MM. 1992: Infection after intramedullary nailing of the tibia. Incidence and protocol for management. *J Bone Joint Surg Br*; **74**: 770–4.
2. Gopal S, Majumder S, Batchelor A, Knight S, Boer PD, Smith R. 2000: Fix and flap: The radical orthopaedic and plastic treatment of severe open fractures of the tibia. *J Bone Joint Surg Br*; **82**: 959–66.

3. Krettek C, Miclau T, Schandelmaier P, Stephan C, Mohlmann U, Tscherne H. 1999: The mechanical effect of blocking screws ("Poller screws") in stabilizing tibia fractures with short proximal or distal fragments after insertion of small-diameter intramedullary nails. *J Orthop Trauma*; **13**: 550–3.
4. Naique SB, Pearse M, Nanchahal J. 2006: Management of severe open tibial fractures: The need for combined Orthopaedic and Plastic Surgical treatment in specialist centres. *J Bone Joint Surg Br*; **88**: 351–7.

18 GUIDELINES FOR PRIMARY AMPUTATION

Principal recommendations

1. A primary amputation is performed as a damage control procedure if there is uncontrollable haemorrhage from the open tibial injury (usually from multiple levels of arterial/venous damage in blast injuries) or for crush injuries exceeding a warm ischaemic period of 6 h.
2. Primary amputation is also needed for incomplete traumatic amputations where the distal remnant is significantly injured.
3. A primary amputation is considered an option where injury characteristics include one or several of the following:
   (a) Avascular limbs exceeding a 4–6 h hour threshold of warm ischaemia
   (b) Segmental muscle loss affecting more than two compartments
   (c) Segmental bone loss greater than one-third of the length of the tibia.
4. Absent or reduced plantar sensation at initial presentation is not an indication for amputation.
5. Amputation levels are preferably transtibial or transfemoral (if salvage of the knee is not possible). Through-knee amputations are not recommended for adults.
6. The decision to amputate primarily should be taken by two consultant surgeons with, if possible, patient and family involvement.
7. Discussion with the nearest specialist centre is advised when there is uncertainty or disagreement between surgeon recommendations and patient/family wishes.

Introduction

A decision to amputate a limb needs to balance the impact of reconstruction and salvage against that of limb removal. The scientific approach, turned to when there are uncertainties in treatment decisions, is unhelpful; a randomized controlled trial is unlikely to get balanced recruitment simply because most patients will not opt to be randomly allocated to amputation if there is a reasonable chance that limb salvage might produce a functional limb.

Modern surgical techniques offer the potential to reconstruct limbs which were thought unsalvageable a few years ago. Vehicle design improvements have also made it more likely that traffic collision victims will survive, albeit with more severe injuries. These factors, combined with occasional episodes of severe blast injuries encountered in civilian practice, mean a surgeon may encounter severe limb trauma that poses the dilemma: should limb salvage be undertaken? Futile attempts to preserve a limb which should be amputated disrupt a patient's life both physically and psychologically. Early amputation can avoid this eventuality but is not without its own problems.[1,2]

Assessment in limb-threatening trauma

Even in the presence of limb-threatening injuries, a firm grasp of the 'big picture' is essential. Advanced Trauma Life Support (ATLS)® management appropriately emphasizes the primary survey as the starting point. Life-threatening problems are identified and treated in a logical, hierarchical sequence. Assessment of limb-threatening trauma is part of the primary survey in 'C' for circulation and 'D' for disability.

A rapid assessment of perfusion, soft tissue injury, fracture pattern and, wherever possible, sensation and motor function is essential. Multiple levels of injury in the same limb pose a difficult problem in assessment – if there is a vascular or neurological deficit, identifying the level of arterial or nerve injury may not be possible from clinical examination alone. Multiple limb trauma will also pose problems. Neurological examination may, at best, be incomplete or even impossible owing to the likelihood of other injuries affecting major systems and rendering the patient unable to respond clearly. In that event, the inability to assess neurology should be clearly documented.

The decision node for amputation against limb salvage is beset with multiple branches. Each branch carries combinations of injury-, patient-, surgeon- and even family-determined variables. Decisions to perform amputations are usually taken at two points in time:[3] (1) immediately, as part of primary treatment or, (2) when either features of the injury or patient recovery declare themselves fully and render any further attempts to save the limb unwise. In the latter group are those cases where initial attempts at salvage fail whilst the patient remains in hospital, as well as those where the family and patient wishes are reflected on.

Immediate amputation is indicated in several open tibial fracture scenarios. These include:

1. Incomplete amputations, where the injury has almost completely severed the limb and the distal portion is itself subject to significant trauma
2. Extensive crush injury, particularly to the foot and distal tibia
3. An avascular limb with a warm ischaemia time in excess of 4 h.

Less certain are scenarios which form the 'grey areas':

1. An ischaemic limb with clinical evidence of nerve dysfunction, particularly absent plantar sensation
2. Segmental muscle loss across more than two compartments, especially if the posterior compartment is involved

3. Segmental bone loss greater than one-third of the length of the tibia
4. Severe open foot injury associated with the tibial fracture.

In addition to the anatomical and functional deficits (which imply the extent of re-construction or repair needed as well as the likely outcome), there needs to be an appreciation of the patient's reserve – physiological, psychological, social and econo-mic. A patient with a 'grey area' scenario with continued haemodynamic instability may shift the decision towards amputation. A patient with a substance abuse history, including alcohol, may struggle to cope with the rigours of protracted limb salvage. Similarly, an individual who is self-employed and a bread-winner needs a predictable and assured period of recovery and may be better served with an amputation. To com-pound matters, the acceptance of limb loss varies greatly between societies of North America and Western Europe, in contrast to the Middle and Far East.

Attempts have been made to produce clinically useful scoring systems to assist in ma-king decisions about limb salvage in these difficult circumstances. However, none has proven useful.[4] Data from the North American Lower Extremity Assessment Project (LEAP) have yielded differences in the priority of limb-threatening variables to am-putation, even amongst experienced trauma surgeons and general trauma surgeons.[3,5,6] A systematic review of the literature[7] showed similar outcomes when comparing am-putation and salvage for grade IIIB and IIIC fractures.

Some idea of the time scale, surgical stages and likely outcome of reconstruction of these scenarios may assist in decision-making. At times, the decision not to amputate immediately is taken in order to gain more information – from the patient and family, or to allow a more complete assessment of the extent of limb injury.

Impact of limb-threatening variables

Limb ischaemia

Warm ischaemia time serves as a threshold as do the extent and levels of associated non-vascular injury in the open fracture (see Chapter 14). The greater the ischaemic time, the more likely it is that there is significant muscle loss from necrosis, no-reflow and reperfusion injury.[8] Salvage of an ischaemic limb in association with an open tibial injury needs to be achieved within 4–6 h if it is to be successful. The 4–6 h warm ischaemia threshold is reduced if the patient is hypotensive throughout most of this time.[9] The use of temporary intravascular shunts can be extremely ef-fective in reducing warm ischaemia time and allows prompt fracture stabilization to proceed before definitive arterial repair.[10] Major deep venous injuries proximal to the trifurcation should also be repaired.[11,12] In the event that the warm ischaemia threshold is approached and the limb is unlikely to receive temporary intravascu-lar shunts immediately, due consideration should be given to amputation. Delayed revascularization may not only induce greater local damage but may also pro-duce systemic effects through the circulation of breakdown products of reperfused muscle.

Absent plantar sensation

It is not uncommon for this clinical finding to exist with evidence of vascular disruption as both nerve and artery course the lower limb together. Absent plantar sensation at initial presentation should not be regarded as an absolute indication for amputation. Recovery of normal plantar sensation is possible in over half the patients and may suggest the initial loss is due to neuropraxia and cannot be assumed to arise from nerve disruption.[5] If structural disruption of the nerve is confirmed during wound assessment, the outcome is less certain, even if the integrity of the nerve is restored by microsurgical repair. Long-term outcomes for patients with permanent absent plantar sensation are unknown, although analogies are made with other non-traumatic conditions which also produce neuropathic feet, e.g. diabetes and spinal cord pathology. An important difference between the insensate traumatic and non-traumatic groups may be the extent of muscle loss and scarring in the former that may influence pain and functional levels; these two groups are not exactly comparable.

Altered plantar sensation requires exploration of the tibial nerve at the time of debridement in open tibial fractures. Structural continuity of the nerve should prompt an expectant approach and not weigh towards a decision for amputation. Conversely, early amputation should be considered if the nerve is found to be divided together with extensive muscle loss across two or more compartments (particularly if the posterior compartment is involved) and a warm ischaemia time greater than 4–6 h. A neuropathic sole with an abnormal, poorly functional foot and ankle are likely outcomes if limb salvage is contemplated in this scenario.

Severe soft tissue damage and loss

The extent and level of muscle loss influence the functional potential in the limb. Muscle damage may occur as a direct consequence of trauma or through effects of ischaemia and reperfusion injury.

Loss of dorsiflexion from anterior compartment loss can be offset by transfer of a functioning tibialis posterior through the interosseous membrane. Loss of peroneal muscle action can be offset by transfer of tibialis posterior to the peroneal tendons behind the tibia. When there is loss of muscle action spanning several compartments, it increases the likelihood of dependence on orthotics to support the foot and ankle. Whilst this alone is not an indication for amputation, other variables often present with the severe soft tissue damage and need to be considered. For example, the presence of extensive muscle damage in the posterior compartment usually is associated with segmental bone loss and disruption of posterior tibial vessels and nerve. Such a combination is seen most frequently after a crush injury and may be an indication for amputation.

Severe bone loss

Bone loss is managed through several strategies: autogenous bone grafts (usually of iliac crest origin), bone substitutes, free vascularized bone or composite tissue transfer and bone regeneration through distraction osteogenesis. A threshold for amputation set by the amount of bone loss is difficult to quantify – cuneiform patterns of bone loss (typically from extrusion of butterfly fragments), even when large, are easily treated with simple autogenous grafts in comparison to segmental patterns of bone loss. Thus, variations exist, not only in the size and type of bone defect, but also in host tissue conditions and the patient's general health.

Guidelines can be obtained by a comparison of the scale and time needed for recovery following salvage when compared to recovery from amputation. In the adult tibia, autogenous bone grafting of segmental defects less than 2 cm in length will consolidate in approximately 5 months, provided the recipient site is well vascularized and the patient is a non-smoker. Larger defects, if treated by distraction osteogenesis, usually consolidate at approximately 45 days per centimetre of tibia replaced. Therefore, a 5 cm defect can be successfully reconstructed using this method in about 7–8 months. However, limb reconstruction using distraction osteogenesis is time consuming and may involve more than one surgical procedure in the period. When segmental bone defects approach 10–15 cm, reconstruction by bone transport will take in excess of 12 months. Only well-motivated patients with appropriate domestic and financial support will be suitable to undertake this magnitude of limb salvage. Free vascularized transfer of bone into the defect (usually the fibula) may shorten the reconstruction time and prove a better alternative, but protection of the transferred bone until suitable hypertrophy occurs is needed in the after-care period.[13,14] In contrast, a transtibial amputee will take approximately 5–6 months to rehabilitate to independent walking if there are no other injuries. In general, bone loss in excess of one-third the length of the tibia will take more than 12 months to reconstruct using distraction osteogenesis. In this situation, amputation should be considered as a viable alternative solution, particularly if the patient has need for early return to independent ambulation and work.

Open foot injuries (in association with open tibial fracture)

This is a segmental injury to the lower limb with special significance: hind-foot injuries are usually complex, and vary from open calcaneal injuries to talar body and neck fractures. In very severe examples, there is extrusion of part of the talus (see Chapter 15).

Whilst the principles of management to both levels of injury are similar, some projection of the likely functional outcome after salvage is needed. Severe hind-foot injuries end up with joint stiffness. Loss of plantar skin is very difficult to reconstruct, even with reinnervated flaps. Salvage of early post-traumatic joint degeneration will need arthrodesis. This sequence of reconstruction and further salvage procedures, should complications within the joints supervene, may leave the patient with the functional equivalent of a below-knee prosthesis. In this event, an early recommendation for a transtibial amputation could provide a functionally equivalent outcome with a shorter rehabilitation period.

Damage control over primary limb salvage

Amputation as damage control

Amputation may serve as the only means for haemorrhage control and resuscitation. Another scenario is a limb that has been crushed for several hours (exceeding the warm ischaemic threshold) and reperfusion may induce severe systemic upset through circulating breakdown products of muscle.

Shunt and span as damage control

When the patient's condition demands a damage control strategy, prolonged surgery to salvage a limb-threatening injury is unhelpful. Damage control orthopaedics in a physiologically unstable patient avoids tipping the patient's inflammatory response into adult respiratory distress syndrome (ARDS), disseminated intravascular coagulation (DIC) and multiple organ failure.[15] A decision has to be made either to amputate the limb or do the minimum to salvage, with a plan to return later for more definitive surgery. The level of temporizing can vary; at its most fundamental, intravascular shunts can be placed for ischaemic limbs and the fracture spanned by external fixation[8] (see Chapter 14). Wound debridement may have to be limited to removal of gross contamination, thereby avoiding extensive exposure and dissection in a coagulopathic patient. The shunts can be left *in situ* whilst the patient remains in the intensive care unit. Shunts with a 'dwell' time averaging 23.5 h have been reported, with a thrombosis rate of 5%.[10] A return for definitive arterial or venous repair coupled to more definitive debridement, should the patient's general condition improve, has to be undertaken at the earliest opportunity or a decision made to amputate. The timing of a return to surgery must be decided upon jointly by the intensive care specialists, plastic and orthopaedic surgical teams.

Amputation levels

The level of amputation is an important consideration with implications for future mobility and employment prospects.[2,16–18] The physical effort of walking is lower and the quality of life superior with a transtibial (below knee) as compared to a transfemoral (above knee) amputation. Energy expenditure for a transtibial amputee is 10–30%[19–21] greater as compared to a 40–67%[20] increase in transfemoral cases. Bilateral transtibial amputees incur an extra energy cost of over 40%, whereas those with bilateral amputations where one level is transfemoral may have to double their energy costs simply to ambulate.[19] The impact of this increased energy cost will vary between patients; in younger, more-able individuals the penalty may not translate into functional significance, but in others both ambulation speed and walking capacity are limited.[20] Similarly, amputees resulting from trauma have lower energy costs compared to those resulting from peripheral vascular disease.[20] Even so, function with modern transtibial prostheses can be excellent and many young patients return to work and sporting activities.

Amputations through the ankle or knee are not recommended for adults. The theoretical advantage of a longer lever arm is not supported by clinical outcomes. Furthermore, patients dislike the pronounced knee level asymmetry (especially when seated) with through-knee amputations. The functional outcome of a through-knee amputation is also poorer to an above-knee equivalent.[2]

Every effort must be made to preserve the knee, including vascular repair or flap coverage, even if the distal limb is hopelessly injured and needs amputating. Very short below-knee amputation stumps can be avoided if, in the presence of a reasonable foot remnant, a pedicled flap of plantar skin and attached os calcis is transferred and fixed to the end of the divided tibia.[22] Such 'partial salvage' can make an enormous difference to ultimate function.

Conclusion

Medium-term studies show comparable outcomes in terms of function, return to work and quality of life for those with successful reconstruction or amputation.[5,23,24] Long-term follow-up of US Army Veterans with lower limb amputations indicate that many people are capable of successful adaptation to their circumstances and lead lives with comparable health-related quality of life to their peers, at least for below-knee amputees.[16–18] Those with transfemoral amputations tended to abandon their prostheses after 10 years or more, opting for mobility in a wheelchair.

Limb salvage is complex and demanding for both patient and surgical team. An amputation should always be considered as an option for open tibial fractures where the severity of injury and patient characteristics shift the balance away from limb salvage. Financial considerations are always quoted as a reason for amputation over limb reconstruction but the sum incurred in a lifetime of prosthesis supply and adjustments can be higher compared to reconstruction in Western societies.[25,26] Furthermore, the ageing amputee can encounter additional problems with mobility that are avoided with successful limb salvage.[27,28]

Wherever possible the decision to amputate should be taken by two consultant surgeons. This serves a dual purpose: reassurance for the patient and their family that a second opinion has been sought, and confirmation (and to some extent protection) for the operating surgeon that such a momentous decision is unavoidable.

References

1. Schoppen T, Boonstra A, Groothoff JW, de Vries J, Goeken LN, Eisma WH. 2003: Physical, mental, and social predictors of functional outcome in unilateral lower-limb amputees. *Arch Phys Med Rehabil*; **84**: 803–11.
2. MacKenzie EJ, Bosse MJ, Castillo RC, *et al*. 2004: Functional outcomes following trauma-related lower-extremity amputation. *J Bone Joint Surg Am*; **86**: 1636–45.
3. MacKenzie EJ, Bosse MJ, Kellam JF, *et al*. 2002: Factors influencing the decision to amputate or reconstruct after high-energy lower extremity trauma. *J Trauma*; **52**: 641–9.

4. Busse JW, Jacobs CL, Swiontkowski MF, Bosse MJ, Bhandari M. 2007: Complex limb salvage or early amputation for severe lower-limb injury: A meta-analysis of observational studies. *J Orthop Trauma*; **21**: 70–6.

5. Bosse MJ, McCarthy ML, Jones AL, *et al*. 2005: The insensate foot following severe lower extremity trauma: An indication for amputation? *J Bone Joint Surg Am*; **87**: 2601–8.

6. Webb LX, Bosse MJ, Castillo RC, MacKenzie EJ. 2007: Analysis of surgeon-controlled variables in the treatment of limb-threatening type-III open tibial diaphyseal fractures. *J Bone Joint Surg Am*; **89**: 923–8.

7. Saddawi-Konefka D, Kim HM, Chung KC. 2008: A systematic review of outcomes and complications of reconstruction and amputation for type IIIB and IIIC fractures of the tibia. *Plast Reconstr Surg*; **122**: 1796–805.

8. Glass GE, Pearse MF, Nanchahal J. 2009: Improving lower limb salvage following fractures with vascular injury: A systematic review and new management algorithm. *J Plast Reconstr Aesthet Surg*; **62**: 571–9.

9. Khalil IM, Livingston DH. 1986: Intravascular shunts in complex lower limb trauma. *J Vasc Surg*; **4**: 582–7.

10. Subramanian A, Vercruysse G, Dente C, Wyrzykowski A, King E, Feliciano DV. 2008: A decade's experience with temporary intravascular shunts at a civilian level I trauma center. *J Trauma*; **65**: 316–24; discussion 324–6.

11. Barros D'Sa AA, Harkin DW, Blair PH, Hood JM, McIlrath E. 2006: The Belfast approach to managing complex lower limb vascular injuries. *Eur J Vasc Endovasc Surg*; **32**: 246–56.

12. Kuralay E, Demirkilic U, Ozal E, *et al*. 2002: A quantitative approach to lower extremity vein repair. *J Vasc Surg*; **36**: 1213–8.

13. Song HR, Kale A, Park HB, *et al*. 2003: Comparison of internal bone transport and vascularized fibular grafting for femoral bone defects. *J Orthop Trauma*; **17**: 203–11.

14. Banic A, Hertel R. 1993: Double vascularized fibulas for reconstruction of large tibial defects. *J Reconstr Microsurg*; **9**: 421–8.

15. Pape HC, Giannoudis PV, Krettek C, Trentz O. 2005: Timing of fixation of major fractures in blunt polytrauma: Role of conventional indicators in clinical decision making. *J Orthop Trauma*; **19**: 551–62.

16. Dougherty PJ. 1999: Long-term follow-up study of bilateral above-the-knee amputees from the Vietnam War. *J Bone Joint Surg Am*; **81**: 1384–90.

17. Dougherty PJ. 2003: Long-term follow-up of unilateral transfemoral amputees from the Vietnam war. *J Trauma*; **54**: 718–23.

18. Dougherty PJ. 2001: Transtibial amputees from the Vietnam War. Twenty-eight-year follow-up. *J Bone Joint Surg Am*; **83**: 383–9.

19. Esquenazi A, Meier RH 3rd. 1996: Rehabilitation in limb deficiency. 4. Limb amputation. *Arch Phys Med Rehabil*; **77** (Suppl): S18–28.

20. Czerniecki JM. 1996: Rehabilitation in limb deficiency. 1. Gait and motion analysis. *Arch Phys Med Rehabil*; **77** (Suppl): S3–8.

21. Mattes SJ, Martin PE, Royer TD. 2000: Walking symmetry and energy cost in persons with unilateral transtibial amputations: matching prosthetic and intact limb inertial properties. *Arch Phys Med Rehabil*; **81**: 561–8.

22. Ghali S, Harris PA, Khan U, Pearse M, Nanchahal J. 2005: Leg length preservation with pedicled fillet of foot flaps after traumatic amputations. *Plast Reconstr Surg*; **115**: 498–505.

23. MacKenzie EJ, Bosse MJ, Pollak AN, *et al*. 2005: Long-term persistence of disability following severe lower-limb trauma. Results of a seven-year follow-up. *J Bone Joint Surg Am*; **87**: 1801–9.

24. Bosse MJ, MacKenzie EJ, Kellam JF, *et al*. 2002: An analysis of outcomes of reconstruction or amputation after leg-threatening injuries. *N Engl J Med*; **347**: 1924–31.

25. Williams MO. 1994: Long-term cost comparison of major limb salvage using the Ilizarov method versus amputation. *Clin Orthop Relat Res*; **301**: 156–8.

26. MacKenzie EJ, Jones AS, Bosse MJ, *et al*. 2007: Health-care costs associated with amputation or reconstruction of a limb-threatening injury. *J Bone Joint Surg Am*; **89**: 1685–92.

27. Brinker MR, O'Connor DP. 2007: Outcomes of tibial nonunion in older adults following treatment using the Ilizarov method. *J Orthop Trauma*; **21**: 634–42.

28. Andrews KL. 1996: Rehabilitation in limb deficiency. 3. The geriatric amputee. *Arch Phys Med Rehabil*; **77** (Suppl): S14–7.

14. Subasi M, Kapukaya A, Arslan H, Ozkul E, Cebesoy O. 2007: Outcome of open comminuted tibial plateau fractures treated using an external fixator. *J Orthop Sci*; **12**: 347–53.
15. Lingard EA, Katz JN, Wright RJ, Wright EA, Sledge CB. 2001: Validity and responsiveness of the Knee Society Clinical Rating System in comparison with the SF-36 and WOMAC. *J Bone Joint Surg Am*; **83**: 1856–64.
16. Khan U, Smitham P, Pearse M, Nanchahal J. 2007: Management of severe open ankle injuries. *Plast Reconstr Surg*; **119**: 578–89.

20 MANAGEMENT OF SEVERE OPEN FRACTURES IN CHILDREN

Principal recommendations

1. The wound for open paediatric fractures is debrided (excised) as recommended for adults. There is no evidence to suggest that tissues with compromised viability are more likely to recover in children compared to adults.
2. Skeletal fixation is determined by the fracture configuration. The use of intramedullary devices may be limited by the presence of growth plates.
3. The available evidence suggests that children under the age of 12 years (prepubertal) are likely to have shorter union times.
4. Soft tissue reconstruction for open fractures in children of all ages relies on vascularized flaps, as it does for adults.

Literature review

A review of the English literature revealed only eight papers[1-8] detailing the management of grade IIIb fractures in children (age < 18 years). These describe a total of 54 open fractures with a mean age of 11 years. The data in these publications have been systematically reviewed by Glass et al.[9]

Timing of debridement following injury

The only series to explore the relationship between time to first operative debridement and infection rate reported that for all paediatric open tibial fractures, the infection rate increased from 12% (two of eight) to 25% (five of 42) when debridement was delayed beyond 6 h.[4] However, a multicentre review of 554 open paediatric fractures found no difference in infection rate where the first debridement was delayed beyond 6 h.[10] The authors proposed a first procedure within 24 h, with antibiotic cover on admission.

Skeletal fixation, union and infection

Techniques for external fixation included unilateral, bi-planar and circular frames. The most common method of open reduction internal fixation used intramedullary nailing. AO plates were used in two of 11 cases reported by Stewart et al and Kirshner wire fixation in another.[8] Buckley et al[1] reported the use of an external fixator with lag screws in one patient. Plaster cast immobilization after removal of external fixator was documented in one series.[3] The use of autogenous bone graft harvested from the iliac crest was documented in seven patients.[1,5,6]

There appeared to be no association between the method of skeletal fixation and union time or with complications, including deep infection and non/malunion.

Twelve of 54 fractures (22%) developed delayed union and seven of 54 (13%) developed non-union. Of the three malunions (all of which occurred following delayed union), two were reported in a publication which did not define the term.[4]

It has been suggested that children younger than 12 years may account for the favourable healing seen among children in general.[11] Jones and Duncan[3] reviewed five grade IIIB tibial fractures in children, with a mean age of 7.6 years. They demonstrated a relatively short mean union time of 18 weeks with external fixation and flap cover and no deep infections. The mean union time for 12 patients under the age of 12 years was 23 weeks (range 12–56 weeks). This was substantially shorter than the mean of 31 weeks (range 5–104 weeks) for the 43 cases of grade IIIB fractures where union times were available.

Infections were subdivided into 'superficial' and 'deep' in seven of the eight series, representing a total of 42 cases. There were five deep infections and seven superficial infections, which most commonly involved external fixator pin sites.

Soft tissue reconstruction

Twenty-eight of 54 grade IIIB fractures were reconstructed using free flaps, 17 with local flaps (16 fasciocutaneous flaps and one local muscle flap) and two were covered by non-specified flaps.[9] One series reported the use of split skin grafting only in four of 10 cases and one patient healed by secondary intention.[1] One publication reported two direct closures.[4] Another fracture was closed as a delayed primary procedure.[7] A further case was closed initially using a skin graft but, following infection and debridement, was subsequently covered with a fasciocutaneous flap.[8]

Of the 28 free flaps, three complications were reported: a thrombosed venous anastomosis, which was successfully revised, loss of 50% of one flap following debridement as a result of partial necrosis, and a rim necrosis.[9] While the sample size was small, these few complications are comparable to figures for adults, where a free flap failure rate of around 2% and a partial failure rate of 6% have been reported following soft tissue reconstruction after lower limb trauma.[12] Of the nine cases which were initially not covered by flaps, five were closed using a split skin graft only, two were closed directly following debridement and skeletal fixation, one had delayed primary closure and one was left to heal by secondary intention.[1,4,7] Three of these nine patients developed deep infection, compared with two of 45 patients (p = 0.028) closed using flap cover. These data suggest improved outcomes in terms of deep infection for Gustilo grade IIIB tibial shaft fractures covered with flaps.

Conclusion

There are few reports regarding grade IIIB tibial fractures in children and evaluation of the data is hampered by a lack of consistency in the application of classifications such as that proposed by Gustilo, the methods used to describe fracture configuration, and the definitions of outcome measures such as union time.

The available data suggest that the time to union, assessed radiologically, may be shorter in children than in adults. Specifically, children younger than 12 years may exhibit faster bone healing. However, Gustilo grade IIIB open fractures can be associated with mal- and non-union, even among young children. Functional outcome data are lacking.

In terms of debridement, the adequacy rather than the timing of debridement appears to be important. There is no evidence to suggest that soft tissues in children are more likely to recover or that lesser procedures, namely skin grafting or allowing wounds to granulate, can substitute for vascularized flap coverage. In fact, attempts to avoid flaps are more likely to result in deep infection. Therefore, the soft tissues in children should be managed as in adults.

References

1. Buckley SL, Smith GR, Spondseller PD, Thompson JD, Robertson WW, Griffin P. 1996: Severe (Type III) open fractures of the tibia in children. *J Pediatr Orthop*; **16**: 627–34.
2. Grimard G, Naudie D, Laberge LC, Hamdy RC. 1996: Open fractures of the tibia in children. *Clin Orthop Relat Res*; **332**: 62–70.
3. Jones BG, Duncan RD. 2003: Open tibial fractures in children under 13 years of age – 10 years experience. *Injury*; **34**: 776–80.
4. Kreder HJ, Armstrong P. 1995: A review of open tibia fractures in children. *J Pediatr Orthop*; **15**: 482–8.
5. Levy AS, Wetzler M, Lewars M, Bromberg J, Spoo J, Whitelaw GP. 1997: The orthopedic and social outcome of open tibia fractures in children. *Orthopedics*; **20**: 593–8.
6. Rinker B, Valerio IL, Stewart DH, Pu LL, Vasconez HC. 2005: Microvascular free flap reconstruction in pediatric lower extremity trauma: A 10-year review. *Plast Reconstr Surg*; **115**: 1618–24.
7. Robertson P, Karol LA, Rab GT. 1996: Open fractures of the tibia and femur in children. *J Pediatr Orthop*; **16**: 621–6.
8. Stewart KJ, Tytherleigh-Strong G, Bharathwaj S, Quaba AA. 1999: The soft tissue management of children's open tibial fractures. *J R Coll Surg Edinb*; **44**: 24–30.
9. Glass GE, Pearse MF, Nanchahal J. 2009: The ortho-plastic management of Gustilo grade IIIB fractures of the tibia in children: A systemic review of the literature and management algorithm. *Injury*; May 4. [Epub ahead of print].
10. Stewart DG Jr, Kay RM, Skaggs DL. 2005: Open fractures in children. Principles of evaluation and management. *J Bone Joint Surg Am*; **87**: 2784–98.
11. Blasier RD, Barnes CL. 1996: Age as a prognostic factor in open tibial fractures in children. *Clin Orthop Relat Res*; **331**: 261–4.
12. Yazar S, Lin CH, Lin YT, Ulusal AE, Wei FC. 2006: Outcome comparison between free muscle and free fasciocutaneous flaps for reconstruction of distal third and ankle traumatic open tibial fractures. *Plast Reconstr Surg*; **117**: 2468–75; discussion 2476–7.

INDEX